D0473660

The
Business Plan
for the
Body

The
Business Plan
for the
Body

CRUNCH THE NUMBERS FOR
SUCCESSFUL WEIGHT LOSS

MANAGE YOUR METABOLISM
BY EATING THE RIGHT WAY

INVEST IN THE ONLY WORKOUT
YOU'LL EVER NEED

JIM KARAS

THREE RIVERS PRESS • NEW YORK

This book proposes a program of physical exercise and dietary recommendations for the reader to follow. However, before starting this or any other exercise program or diet regimen, you should consult your physician.

Copyright © 2001 by Jim Karas

All rights reserved. No part of this book may be reproduced or transmitted in any form or by any means, electronic or mechanical, including photocopying, recording, or by any information storage and retrieval system, without permission in writing from the publisher.

Published by Three Rivers Press, New York, New York. Member of the Crown Publishing Group.

Random House, Inc. New York, Toronto, London, Sydney, Auckland

www.randomhouse.com

THREE RIVERS PRESS is a registered trademark and the Three Rivers Press colophon is a trademark of Random House, Inc.

Design by Elina D. Nudelman

Printed in the United States of America

Library of Congress Cataloging-in-Publication Data
Karas, Jim.
    The business plan for the body : crunch the numbers for successful weight loss*manage your metabolism by eating the right way*invest in the only workout you'll ever need / by Jim Karas.—1st ed.
        p. cm.
    Includes index.
    1. Weight loss.   I. Title.
RM222.2 .K337 2001
613.2'5—dc21   00-051224

ISBN 0-609-80742-0

10 9

To my daughter, Olivia, who, as she grows, reinforces my belief that if you apply yourself, anything is possible.

ACKNOWLEDGMENTS

While there are numerous people to thank for the encouragement and support I received during the planning and writing of this book, four in particular need to be singled out. The first two, Patti Salvagio and Robert Lang, I lovingly refer to as my "country club" staff. I call them this since neither really needs the job nor the aggravation, but both come to work, in between vacations and personal services, maybe a little later than most, and help me run my firm, Solo Sessions.

Patti, my business manager, brings a wonderful energy to the organization and puts up with never-ending schedule changes, phone calls, and some behavioral problems, which are frequently displayed. We both share the belief that people come into each other's lives for a reason. I am lucky she came into mine.

Robert Lang does all the marketing and public relations for my firm, helped me write my book proposal, and gave considerable form and shape to this book. He is also my daughter's godfather and my best friend. Bob is my sounding board and gives me the confidence to never stop trying. Together, the three of us spend hours every week together. They put up with my sophomoric humor, my dictatorial managerial style, and, occasionally, a few tears. I could not have completed this project without them.

Next is my wife, Ellen. Juggling her own career (she is an actress), our home, daughter, and son, plus the demands of my work is not an easy task. I appreciate the support and the love that she gives me on a daily basis. I know I'm not always easy to be around at times. Just know I'm trying.

Finally, my daughter Olivia. Since the day four years ago when she came on the scene, my life has never been the same. She is my inspiration. The time we spend together, whether playing house, Candy Land and king and princess, fast dancing, eating cookie pretzels or our regular lunches on Saturday and Sunday, is the best. I loved the times when I was writing at home and she would sit on my lap and ask to play on my "umputer." I would watch her pound on the keyboard in utter amazement that she is a part of me and a part of my life. This book is for you, Olivia. I hope it helps pay for a little private schooling.

CONTENTS

The
Business Plan
for the
Body

INTRODUCTION

Dick Walsh, one of my favorite clients, a friend, and a very successful businessman, once told me "the world gets out of the way for a man with a plan." I believe that to be true. Dick and Yogi had a plan, they achieved success. If you are presently unhappy with your weight, health, and appearance, I am going to make an assumption: You lack a plan. Do you look at your schedule every week and block out time for exercise? Do you shop in advance, think about when and what you are going to eat? Do you steer friends and business associates to restaurants where you know you can get a healthy, low-calorie meal? Let's face it, you probably don't do any of these. You don't have a real plan, but the fact that you have this book in your hand indicates you do have a desire. To satisfy this desire, you must act. You need *The Business Plan for the Body*.

The Business Plan for the Body is the first book to apply the concepts of a business plan to a successful weight-loss strategy. Business plan, weight loss, how do the two come together? I graduated from the University of Pennsylvania's Wharton School in May 1983 with a bachelor of science degree in economics. Armed with my diploma, I was determined to become the next Blake Carrington. Remember the popular 1980s television show *Dynasty*? After all, Blake was a self-made millionaire, had been married to Joan Collins and was presently married to Linda

"If you don't know where you're going, you'll end up somewhere else...."

YOGI BERRA

Evans, lived in a mansion, and tooled around in private planes and chauffeur-driven limousines. Very eighties, but it worked for me. My first job landed me on the Chicago Board Options Exchange, where I found myself working for Merrill Lynch, waving and screaming like a crazy person all day on the trading floor. From there, on to New York City and a stint as the assistant to the president and editor in chief of *Leaders* magazine. For a year I traveled around the world, interviewed and met celebrities such as former Philippine first lady Imelda Marcos, former president Jimmy Carter, the Dalai Lama of Tibet, hotel magnate Leona Helmsley, clothing designer Bernard Lanvin, former Soviet ambassador Anatoly Dobrynin, Senator Jay Rockefeller, and many others. From there, back to Chicago for a few years as a private portfolio manager. Then, in 1988, I became one of the first personal fitness trainers in Chicago, and went on to build my very successful personal fitness training firm, Solo Sessions.

How did such a drastic career change occur? I was regularly taking an aerobics class in the suburbs of Chicago, and one Saturday morning the teacher failed to appear. About one hundred people were standing in the room trying to decide what to do. I asked one of the staff if she had any of the class music tapes, she said yes, so I said I would teach. I taught the 8:00 A.M. class, and since the teacher still didn't show, the 9:00 A.M. class as well. Afterward, the manager of the club approached me and inquired if I wanted to be a part-time instructor. I was pleased they liked my work. I then asked what the compensation would be. He said four dollars per hour and a free membership. Not exactly the type of numbers I was used to seeing in the world of private finance. But I enjoyed teaching the class, so I figured, "What the hell." I took the offer.

I started teaching part-time and ultimately moved to a club in the city. One day I was approached after the class by one of my more colorful students, who happened to be from Beverly Hills. She asked me if I would work with her one-on-one during the day since it was hard for her to make it to class at the designated times. I said I would think about it. She said she would pay me thirty dollars per hour. She was my first client. Thank you, Janet.

From there my clientele rapidly grew. Realizing I could definitely make a living in this new world, I decided to quit my job in finance and devote myself full-time to fitness. Those who didn't quite get my career switch would cynically ask me, "So what are you doing now?" I would answer, "I'm an aerobics instructor and a personal fitness trainer." Because back then the concept of "personal training" was still new, they would ask me what that meant. I would tell them that I met with clients and worked out with them one-on-one. They began to understand. The word got out.

I have always believed that service should be commensurate with price. So I decided to use some of the knowledge I had acquired through my business school education and become the most expensive personal fitness trainer in the market and provide the highest level of service. It worked. Positioning.

In 1993, I also began a firm called At Home Chef. As I was fitness training and preaching the need to embrace a low-calorie eating regime in order to lose weight, numerous clients, exasperated with my constant references to this low-calorie, healthy eating, said, "Stop talking about the healthy food. Just get it in my house." So I hired a group of chefs who literally go into client's homes and prepare customized low-calorie, tasty, healthy food. Consequently, I now provide my clients with both intelligent fitness training *and* the right eating program to achieve weight loss.

A few years ago I introduced a program called "The $10,000-a-Week Weight-Loss Solution." It started when one of my regular clients said to me during a training session, "If only you could live with me for a week and make me do it. Then I could really get a jump start on my program." So I did. I literally began moving in with clients and acting as a "turnaround specialist" to reverse their weight-gain trend. I fitness-train clients as much as possible, educate them on eating and the caloric value of foods, meet with their spouse, executive assistant, chef, friends, other business associates, whoever the clients and I determine is an integral part of their life (see Chapter 4, "The Management Team"). I design and equip an exercise room, go to the clients' favorite restaurants, and teach them how to maneuver the menu, waiter, and chef. I explore every aspect of the clients' life and identify what has been keeping them from achieving success, including checking their garbage and looking for candy wrappers hidden under their bed. After one week I leave the client with a custom-designed, comprehensive formula for success.

Before long I realized that my approach with these clients was similar to that of a classic business plan. I must have been applying many of the concepts I learned at business school to weight loss. I found myself actually using business analogies with my clients, such as equating revenues, minus expenses, equals profits; to calories in, minus calories out, equals body weight. Suddenly they understood and could relate this concept to weight loss. No gimmicks, crazy strategies, it's just numbers. They saw that weight loss is basically a numerical equation: calories in minus calories out.

Next I did some research. I looked at successful business plans, co-opted the structure and concepts, and applied them to a strategy to achieve weight loss. Then I began writing this book.

Keep in mind, my clients had been paying upward of $10,000 for a week, plus expenses, for my expertise. Clearly, only a small portion of the population can afford this sum. So I thought, why not share this information, and provide many people with the same information for a price considerably less?

The first chapters of the book are the research and development phase of your plan. Business plans traditionally start with a "Mission Statement," so that is Chapter 1. Companies research "The Competition" in their industry; I did that for you in Chapter 2. In Chapter 3, "Going Public," I urge you to be open, honest, and publicize—something few people do—your intention to go into the weight-loss business. Chapter 4, "The Management Team," discusses the importance of educating and including those around you in the development and administration of your plan. "The Financials," Chapter 5, presents the reality of weight loss by the numbers.

Following the R&D phase, you enter into the actual execution of the plan. You implement a proper combination of eating and exercise, Chapter 6, "Revenue Allocation," and Chapter 7, "Preservation of Capital," to facilitate weight loss. Chapter 8, "Establishing Realistic Investment Goals," encourages you to set weight-loss goals that can be attained.

With your plan in action, you move to Chapter 9, "It's Starting to Work: Taking It on the Road; Keeping It Going," which explores changing environments and introduces the concept of "progression." Just as investors continue to modify their portfolio as the financial markets change, a successful weight-loss program requires modification and progression. Specific strategies are discussed to enable an individual to successfully manage change. The plan concludes with Chapter 10, "I Did It, I Did It," which prepares you to live with your success, both physically and emotionally.

This is a journey—a journey guaranteed to facilitate change. Change is difficult. Consequently, there undoubtedly will be moments when you question the wisdom of such a journey. You may even want to give up, rip open a bag of chips or cookies and say the hell with it. But the next day, the scale, the too tight clothing, all those mirrors, the shortness of breath—not to mention all the wonderful aspects of your life that you don't want to leave prematurely—will still be a voice in your head telling you that you must change. *The Business Plan for the Body* is the way to accomplish that transformation. This book gives you a map, guiding you through all aspects of weight loss. No longer will you haphazardly try to do it on your own. Sometimes you will laugh, sometimes you will cry, sometimes you will doubt. Often times you will find the answer to many questions, concerns, and concepts you have never understood or misunderstood. This time, you are going to approach weight loss with your eyes open. No more shooting in the dark.

Since becoming a fitness professional, I have observed, assisted, and at times even been accosted by hundreds, possibly thousands, of people trying to lose weight. Each person would regale me with their "new" diet, "new" medication, or "new" simple solution to what I consider to be a very serious problem. According to James O. Hill, chairman of the World Health Organization's committee on obesity, and president of the North American Association for the Study of Obesity, America is the "world leader" when it comes to being overweight. We are literally the largest nation in the Western world, weighing on average sixteen pounds more than our neighbors in western Europe. We're creating a health crisis, we're aging before our time, we're stressing our bodies inside and out, and we just don't feel as good as we should—despite the fact that we live in the most prosperous nation on earth. Indeed, carrying around extra weight is a serious problem—and one that has to be addressed with a comprehensive plan, not a quick fix! If you're reading this book, that means you're ready for a weight-loss program that offers an intelligent, workable solution with results that will last a lifetime.

With this book, like Yogi and my friend Dick, you, too, will have a plan. You will have *The Business Plan for the Body*—and you will succeed!

Current Market Conditions

PART

I

THE MISSION STATEMENT

1 *What You Want*

I have conducted over five hundred new client meetings during the past thirteen years. I can immediately tell if clients are going to succeed on my program by their body language and the first words out of their mouth. Some people wiggle in their chair, like a truant child in the principal's office, look away and say, "I think I should do something about my situation" or "My doctor told me I have to start a program" or "My friend said I should call you." This tells me they are not committed to succeed. The motivation is not there. The desire is not strong.

Others sit straight up, look me in the eye and say, "That's it. I have had it looking and feeling this way. I want to get a handle on this situation. Tell me what I have to do to lose weight and get in shape. I'm ready." This I love. I know I have someone who is ready to meet the challenge, because, let's face it, taking control of your health and appearance is going to take time, commitment, energy, and focus.

Which individual are you?

So, you're considering getting into the weight-loss business? Allow me to make the following assumption. Along with millions of other people, you have previously attempted this business venture. I will also assume, since you purchased this book, or happen to have it in your hands, that you have not been happy with your previous level of success. Or, perhaps it's as simple as:

> **"Whenever you see a successful business, someone once made a courageous decision."**
>
> **PETER DRUCKER**

- *You walked by a mirror in a department store and wondered who that was wearing the same outfit you had on, or*
- *You bumped into a high school or college friend who didn't recognize you, or*
- *You are convinced your clothes are shrinking, or*
- *You stopped weighing yourself out of fear, or*
- *You feel awful all the time and have no energy, or*
- *Your doctor scared the hell out of you.*

These are just a few of the responses I have heard over the years, but the point remains, *you feel out of control and want help.*

From now on your situation will not be out of control. As many friends and clients will tell you, I do not readily accept defeat. Nor will you. The word "tenacious" has been used to describe me. I want that same word to be used to describe you and your new business venture. I have had thirteen years of experience helping hundreds of people lose weight. I never believe a client will fail. I only believe in success. Each success story, similar to the opening comments to this chapter, has one identical element. The individual looked at me and, in so many words, said, "I want to be in the weight-loss business. I want to succeed at losing weight."

Now I know each and every one of you is saying, "Yeah, I want to lose weight, doesn't everyone?" Yes, many individuals do want to lose weight, but I would venture to say that many individuals would also like to be rich, beautiful (though you may notice, the vast majority of these so-called beautiful people are generally in better shape than most), and celebrated. I can't help you be rich, beautiful, and celebrated, but I will help you to lose weight, which will improve your self-esteem and could actually make you richer, more attractive, and perhaps more celebrated, at least by yourself and those around you. And most likely it can even extend your time on this planet. *The Business Plan for the Body* is the key to weight loss because it is a comprehensive approach that addresses:

The Three Variables to Weight Loss: Eating, Exercise, and the Right Mind-set

The model of a successful business plan can be used to create a strategy for you to lose weight and keep it off once and for all. My plan works.

According to the Food and Drug Administration, as many as 85 percent of dieters put the weight back on within two years after weight loss. Personally, I think this percentage may be higher. And we all know, an overwhelming percentage of new businesses fail as well. Armed with *The Business Plan for the Body,* you will not fail. Why are we overweight? Why aren't we succeeding at weight loss? Why do so many new businesses fail? What is the problem? I believe the problem, and the answer to these questions, begins with the absence of a plan. Most people, and many businesses, fail to go through the necessary steps to conceptualize, formulate, and then implement a strategic plan. Planning is everything. Do you think Bill Gates one day said, "I would like to kinda, sorta, do something with computers?" Or did Martha Stewart say, "I think I throw a halfway decent dinner party. Maybe I can teach other people how to do the same." No. They both probably said or thought something to the effect of, "I know a lot about how to use this new device called a computer," or "I know a lot about home entertaining. I can do it better than my competitors. I know I can create a business out of this knowledge and these skills; I am going to create a business plan." They created not only a goal, but a strategy for achieving that goal. Let me repeat: They created not only a goal but a *strategy* for achieving that goal. In other words, a comprehensive plan for success. I know your goal is weight loss, but have you ever had a comprehensive strategy to achieve that goal? You will now.

WHAT IS A MISSION STATEMENT?

Traditionally, a mission statement begins the business plan. It's a sentence, phrase, or paragraph that describes the ultimate goal of a new or existing business. The basis of your mission statement should be the following sentence: "I am in the weight-loss business." Now, take that mission statement and make it your own. Describe your ultimate fitness and weight-loss goals. Be as specific as you desire. Above all be realistic. Don't try to lose ten pounds in ten days. Don't plan to make the

Olympic swim team if you haven't done a single lap in years. Just be honest about what you want to do for your body and pick a time frame that makes sense.

In Chapter 8, "Establishing Realistic Investment Goals," I urge you to set realistic, attainable fitness and weight-loss goals by the numbers, but for now, personalize your mission statement to make it more powerful to you. For example:

> **"I am in the weight-loss business. I intend to lose all the weight I gained after the birth of my last child."**

> **"I am in the weight-loss business. I want to compete in a triathlon by next fall."**

> **"I am in the weight-loss business. I want to be able to fit into my favorite jeans by my next birthday."**

Write down your mission statement and put it somewhere—paste it in your day planner or the top drawer of your desk—anywhere you will read it regularly. You can revise your mission statement if you need to, but the idea is to pick a goal, stick with it, and reach it. Like any company that is opening its doors for business, you have a mission—and that mission is to succeed.

Look at other successful business entities. What is McDonald's mission statement? Its vision is to be the world's best quick service restaurant experience. How about Southwest Airlines? Its mission is dedication to the highest quality of customer service delivered with a sense of warmth, friendliness, individual pride, and company spirit. The Four Seasons Hotel Group? I would venture to say its mission statement is to provide prestige accommodations, superior dining, and luxury service. These businesses state their goal(s) in straightforward, noncomplicated terms. That is what I am asking you to do.

In the past, as harsh as this may sound, you have been in the *weight-gain* business. Like millions of Americans, who are estimated to spend between thirty to fifty billion dollars a year on weight loss, you have overeaten and underexercised and intermittently tried some quick-fix program to lose weight. Now you are getting out of that business and starting a new one; the *weight-loss business*. Repeat that with me. *You are getting out of the weight-gain business and starting the weight-loss busi-*

ness. Believing in that phrase is the first essential step to building the plan.

I first uttered that phrase in the spring of 1982. I decided to take control of my health and appearance in my early twenties when I was in college. At the time, I was about twenty pounds overweight, had never lifted a weight, and called smoking my "sport." I was studying during the second semester of my junior year at the London School of Economics and decided I was going to stop smoking and get my body in shape. I rented a flat in South Kensington with nonsmoking roommates, who told me under no circumstances was I to smoke anywhere in the flat. I told them that I was going to quit smoking and start exercising. They rolled their eyes.

Well, I quit smoking, but was terrified about gaining weight, which I had done during past attempts. So, in my Tretorn tennis shoes, I started running through Hyde Park and Kensington Gardens in order to get some weight off and feel better. I began in the winter of 1982, a time when the British were not used to seeing young men running in the parks. Most Londoners clutched their children as I lumbered by.

It was hard, but I was determined. It was amazing how quickly I started to feel better. That was nineteen years ago. I have stayed committed, and quickly expanded my program to include strength and resistance training. I feel that once you taste success and look and feel so much better, there is really no turning back. I realize I was young when I made this decision, but studies repeatedly show that benefits will accrue almost immediately, regardless of age. I know the same can happen to you—and keep in mind, I am not one of those people who has never had to lose weight. I struggle with it all the time!

You'll be interested to know that I almost did not graduate from high school because I blew off so many gym classes. I had to go twice a day for one week in order to receive the credit to graduate. Think about it, the "$10,000-a-Week Fitness Trainer" almost flunked gym in high school and had absolutely no interest in exercise. Strange things can happen. I changed, and so can you. Change is difficult. *The Business Plan for the Body* is your guide to coping with that change.

Right now, I bet you are thinking of the time, energy, and emotion involved in getting into the weight-loss business. I won't deny that your new business will require effort on your part. According to internationally known hairstylist and entrepreneur, Vidal Sassoon, "The only place where *success* comes before hard *work* is in the dictionary." Let me provide you with an estimate of the time involved. You will need about five minutes each day to plan your meals. You will need to shop for groceries, which, with the luxury of the phone, fax machines, and the Internet, does not need to take more than a few minutes. With regard to exercise, you will need to block out between two to three hours a week. That can easily be accomplished. I will show you in Chapter 7 how you can succeed at weight loss with the right exercise prescription, time allotment, and duration. It's not as much time as you think, if you apply yourself correctly.

In addition to weight loss, you also derive these additional physical and psychological benefits from following a comprehensive program:

- *Reduction of the risk of cardiovascular disease, cancer, stroke, Type II diabetes, high blood pressure, high cholesterol, osteoporosis, arthritis, gallstones, and gout*
- *Increased blood flow to the brain, which boosts energy level, productivity, creativity, and memory*
- *Reduction of stress and depression*
- *Significant slowing of the aging process.*

You decide. On the one hand you can look better, feel better, slow the aging process, boost your energy, productivity, memory level, and decrease stress and depression. On the other hand, you can stay the way you presently are.

This is your choice, no one else can make it happen. In January 2000, *Consumer Reports on Health* included the results of a survey conducted by dietitian Anne Fletcher, who interviewed 160 people who had successfully kept off the weight they'd set out to lose. Many of the dieters reported that they'd tried numerous methods of weight loss before they were successful. "What distinguished their last, successful attempt was a proverbial 'flip of the switch' in which the desire to lose finally became more important than the desire to overeat or to not exercise." I couldn't agree more. As I pointed out, I can instantly tell by body language if a new client is really interested in getting into the weight-loss business or simply flirting with the idea. Only you can "flip the switch," which, interestingly, is an expression I have been using for years. It is the perfect metaphor because—please forget dimmer switches—either the light is on or off. Either you are on program or off. Halfway is no way. Period.

Since many people know that I am in the fitness industry, I often receive one of two responses when I am introduced socially. They either say, "Hey, I've heard of you. You're in the fitness business. I've thought of starting a weight-loss program. Could you give me your card. I'll give you a call." In the embryonic stages of my fitness career, I would anxiously await their call the following day. It practically never occurred. Frequently, when I would bump into the person, I would casually inquire, "Are you ready yet?" Most would politely say, "Oh yes, I'll give you a call tomorrow." It still never happened.

FLIP THE SWITCH

Then, one day out of the blue, usually on my voice mail at an odd hour, the person would call me and say, "This is a message for Jim Karas. We've met a few times. I need to talk to him today. Could you please have him call me at my home between 7:00 A.M. and 9:00 A.M. or my office between 9:30 A.M. and 6:00 P.M. I am really anxious to get started." I've learned that something happened to this person. In other words, the "switch flipped on." I don't believe they were lying in the past when they said they were interested in a program; they weren't ready or able to act on their desire. Once that call comes in, I know I have a committed, focused, ready to "get to work" client on my hands. Now they are ready. These are the people who succeed and make it a joy to be in my business. It is very gratifying to see someone succeed, and it is a nice feeling to have helped him or her in the process.

Remember, I said that I receive one of two responses from people. Here is the second: I am introduced. I receive the none-too-polite "Hello" or "Hi" as they look the other way. Some people actually go out of their way to be rude and dismissive. I know they know who I am and what I do for a living. "Is it me?" I used to wonder. "Did I do something to offend them?" The answer is no, but yes as well, because I represent their Achilles' heel. I represent their failure. These people can't get their weight, health, and appearance under control, and for some reason, possibly known only to their analyst, they view me as judging them.

An individual's decision to go into the weight-loss business is a very emotional process. While I'm no psychiatrist, I can say that thirteen years of listening to people express their fears and desires in the areas of health and weight, as well as my own experience with weight loss, has provided me with a good deal of data on the subject. Frequently, for my clients, overeating seems to be masking some other issue. These issues, too, should be explored. You can do this on your own or with a professional therapist.

Stop a second. Is this the right time for you to go into the weight-loss business? Maybe yes, maybe no. Take the time to decide. If you need to set aside this book and the idea of going into the weight-loss business, then do it. If this is not an opportune time to undertake this **IS THIS THE RIGHT TIME TO BEGIN?** endeavor, then wait. Put the book by your bed, or in a bookcase next to your television or computer screen. Shelve the book, take an assessment of your mental health, but don't shelve the desire. You might even reread chapters of this book on a regular basis to keep the concepts fresh in your head. Just make sure that when you *do* want to go into the weight-loss business, you have the time, energy, clarity, and focus to turn that desire into a reality.

Remember the 1960s television series *Mission Impossible,* and the recent movies of the same name? The main character, Jim Phelps and Ethan Hunt, played by Peter Graves and Tom Cruise, respectively, would listen to a tape recorder that would say, "Your mission, should you choose to accept it, is . . ." Then the tape would self-destruct in five seconds. Well, this book will not self-destruct, but your body and health will if you don't take control of it.

STRATEGIC ACTION PLAN

Successful business ventures start with a mission statement.

- *Make the choice to create and accept your own personal mission statement.*

The Business Plan for the Body

- *Make the choice to be in the weight-loss business.*
- *Make the choice to reach your goals.*

And most of all, make an intelligent choice about weight loss. Lose weight, feel great, and commit to your new plan, *The Business Plan for the Body.*

2

Who's Getting It Right, Who's Getting It Wrong

A talk show recently had an author discussing how "bad" broccoli was for you because it has a high "something" index. Now stop a moment and think this through with me. Broccoli, one of the most nutritious foods, loaded with vitamins and minerals, packed with fiber and water, and a "whopping" twenty-four calories a cup, is singled out as the reason an individual is overweight? I don't think so. But I promise you, someone out there who is trying to lose weight is going to cut back on his or her broccoli consumption and expect results. Do you think the overeating of broccoli is the reason that over 55 percent of all Americans are overweight? When was the last time friends or coworkers told you how they really blew their diet with broccoli? Did you stay up last night watching late-night television with a huge bowl of broccoli?

> "I haven't failed. I've found ten thousand ways that don't work."
>
> **THOMAS EDISON**

You have decided to go into the weight-loss business. As an astute businessperson, you realize the benefit of researching "the competition," especially when launching a new business venture. Smart investors take the time to look at the current competition, assess their strengths and weaknesses, and use that information to fine-tune their plan. Take the coffee business as an example. As recently as seven years ago, most of the current names such as Starbucks, Seattle's Best Coffee, Caribou Coffee, and the like did not exist nationally. Starbucks was the first to go national, and did so successfully. Many imitators quickly followed suit. I live in downtown Chicago and have watched many of these copycats come and go. In my opinion, they did not fully assess the current market situation or simply tried to duplicate the Starbucks model. The competition incorrectly assumed there was either an unlimited supply of coffee drinkers or consumers would willingly switch brands. Even Starbucks has branched out to add sandwiches and other items to its core product, coffee. Had more analysis been conducted, many if not most of these mistakes could have been avoided.

Millions of Americans have attempted to lose weight. They have tried all sorts of nutty programs. They failed. I have personally "Scarsdaled," "Miracle Souped," "Fasted," and "Food Combined." This time we are going to be smart. We are going to assess the competition and determine who's getting it right, who's getting it wrong, and why.

CURRENT DIETS IN THE MARKETPLACE

High protein diets have recently been all the rage. These programs originated in the 1960s as the Atkins diet, were repackaged in the 1970s as the Stillman diet, once again in the 1980s as the Scarsdale diet, and now here we are in the twenty-first century back to the Atkins diet. They all urge you to exclusively eat meat, cheese, eggs, bacon, butter, and similar high-protein and high-fat foods. They ask you to eliminate almost all carbohydrates, including fruits and vegetables, from your diet. These diets ignore the fact that the high consumption of meat, cheese, and other high fat content foods is condemned by virtually all legitimate medical experts. According to the research published in the *University of California at Berkeley Wellness Newsletter*, high-protein diets are associated with an increased risk of heart disease, some cancers (such as colon and prostate), osteoporosis, and kidney damage. The Berkeley newsletter cites a Harvard study of 86,000 female nurses: The women in the study who ate the most animal protein had 22 percent more forearm fractures (a sign of accelerated osteoporosis). The reason? As your protein intake rises, you tend to lose calcium. Other studies have linked high protein consumption to damage of the liver and immune system. In addition, the majority of these diets do not reduce your intake of saturated fat, which any reputable medical specialist will tell you is a killer.

What these diets do is place the body in a state of ketosis, which forces the body to burn fat for fuel. In the absence of carbohydrates, your body does not burn fat completely and substances called ketones are formed and released into your bloodstream. You may think, "But I want to burn fat for fuel." That's right, and you frequently do so without resorting to this drastic program that places your body in this unhealthy state. Ketosis can also cause you to have vile breath, headaches, sleep problems, nausea, diarrhea, and fatigue. I encountered a man at a party who regaled me with how effective his high-protein diet was. His breath could have removed wallpaper. I felt like I was in a cartoon where the black smoke, or bad breath, kept coming at me. (To make matters worse, this man was like the "close talker" character on *Seinfeld,* and was standing approximately four inches from my face. Not pleasant.)

Undoubtedly, these diets do have appeal because they initially cause the scale to drop. But the weight loss is a reflection of a dramatic loss of body fluids, not fat. These diets, as you may have expected, do advocate reduced caloric consumption. They are not directly telling you this, but yes, these diets are low in calories, which, combined with fluid loss, is the principal reason you lose weight. Ketosis kills your appetite, but mostly because it makes you feel sick. You might be interested to know that the brain is fueled by carbohydrates; so, does eliminating your brain's fuel make sense to you? In addition, these diets severely restrict vitamins and minerals, since they prohibit most fruits and vegetables. Most of these diets even admit this point; consequently, many of them urge you to purchase *their* vitamin supplement.

VEGETABLES AND FRUIT ARE THE KEY

Throughout this book you will hear me sing the praises of vegetables and fruit. You will learn that they should be the majority of what you eat. You will also learn that vegetables and fruit can reduce your risk of heart disease, cancer, stroke, Type II diabetes, and on and on and on. In addition, it has been proven that they can contribute to the slowing of the aging process. Does it make sense to go on a diet that eliminates these foods? Obviously not.

One last health note on high-protein diets: As research has shown, high consumption of animal flesh coupled with low consumption of fruits and vegetables can lead to a buildup of toxins in the colon and an increased risk of often fatal colon cancer, plus, as you can imagine, numerous other gastrointestinal side effects.

Food combining, as in not combining certain foods, continues to be popular. This theory advocates that individuals should not be eating proteins and carbohydrates in the same meal, nor should an individual ever eat fruit with any other food. According to its proponents, by not combining carbohydrates and proteins in the same meal, you restructure your metabolism and lose weight. Unfortunately, there is not a single shred of evidence that supports this theory. Years ago I attempted a similar program and told my doctor about it. I explained that when you eat carbohydrates, one group of enzymes is released by the stomach to digest the food, and when you eat protein, another group of enzymes is sent in to do "the work." If I were to eat a meal that included both proteins and carbohydrates, I would confuse my digestive process and wreak havoc with my metabolism. I know this sounds silly, but I was desperate to lose weight. Upon hearing my explanation, my doctor looked at me and replied, "Are you kidding? That is totally untrue. Where did you hear this nonsense?" Believe me, the so-called concept known as Food Combining contributes nothing to weight loss.

The 40, 30, 30 plan instructs people to eat a daily diet of 40 percent carbohydrates, 30 percent protein, and 30 percent fat. This plan is best known as the basis of the best-selling "Zone" books. The individuals promoting these diet programs claim that eating within these parameters will help your body reach a metabolic state that will keep you thin. How do the experts feel about this? For starters, four respected professional organizations, the American College of Sports Medicine, the American Dietetic Association, the Women's Sports Foundation, and the Cooper Institute for Aerobics Research, released a joint statement saying that "these plans are neither the answer for weight loss nor for athletic performance and can cause harm." *The International Journal of Sports Nutrition* says that the "promises in these books are an appalling oversimplification of complex physiological processes." Does this sound like a wise strategy to you? These experts don't think so, nor do I.

Again, the only reason this program keeps you thin is because the total caloric intake on a daily basis is around 900 calories. Yes, we'd all be thin if we only ate 900 calories daily, but this would compromise our health and promote loss of lean muscle tissue, which you will learn in subsequent chapters is the most active and important tissue in the body to facilitate weight loss. And let's face it, who can stay on a plan of only 900 calories? No one I know. Does eating 40-30-30 matter? No, and once again, there is no case study or evidence to support it. A much more intelligent plan would be higher in carbohydrates, say 55 to 60 percent, and lower in protein and fat, to around 20 percent, respectively. When chronically obese patients in a study done by the University of Vermont lowered their fat intake to about 20 percent of their total calories, they lost an average of twenty to thirty pounds over the course of one year.

Programs that claim that sugar is the culprit have been proven invalid as well. Sugar itself is not the problem, it is the amount of sugar that Americans consume, much of it hidden in prepared foods and drinks, including those products sold as "low fat" or "healthy." Sugar consumption in the United States has increased 28 percent since 1983. Manufacturers took the fat out of food and increased the sugar to give it flavor. Marion Nestle, Ph.D., MPH, chair of the Department of Nutrition and Food Studies at New York University, says, "More sugar means more calories, and more calories means weight gain. Add to that, 43 percent of our sugar intake comes from drinks." We will explore in subsequent chapters the *evil* of liquid calories.

Some very popular diet plans go so far as to claim that any sugar in our diet is a problem. *Tufts University Health & Nutrition Letter* (August 19, 1998) states that "anti-sugar diets present one false claim after another. For example, these programs imply that sugar causes diabetes (it doesn't); that it's a risk factor for heart disease (it isn't); and that the hormone insulin causes weight gain (it won't)." I think the *Tufts Letter* put that beautifully. Enough said.

So, once again, sugar itself is not the problem. It is Americans' huge sugar consumption, which means more calories in. Go back to the equation, calories in minus calories out, described in the introduction. The average U.S. woman has added twenty-seven pounds of sugar, corn syrup, and other high-calorie sweeteners to her annual intake since 1986. Common sense dictates that such excessive consumption is the reason for weight gain more than the sugar itself.

A body type or blood type program claims that individuals with different body or blood types should be on a specific program tailored to their body or blood type. Think about this. According to this theory, if two women, both age fifty, five feet five inches tall, 140 pounds, want to lose weight, then one, say with type A blood, should go on one plan, and the other, with type B, should be on another. Does this sound as crazy to you as it does to me? Or, if one of these women is considered "athletic" while the other is considered "soft," they should go on two different programs. Neither blood type nor body type has anything to do with weight loss. Creating a caloric deficit by eating right and exercising does. Even one of the advocates of this theory, naturopath Peter D'Adamo, author of *Eat Right for Your Type,* was forced to admit that no large studies on the blood type theory have ever been conducted.

Severely restrictive fat intake programs are really only for that special population of individuals with heart disease, or possibly cancer. This type of program was originally designed by Nathan Pritikin, author of countless books such as *The Pritikin Program for Diet & Exercise,* and is very similar to the program developed and researched by Dean Ornish, M.D., also an author of numerous books on this topic, such as *Reversing Heart Disease.* Both Pritikin and Ornish firmly believe that a vegetarian diet consisting of only 10 percent calories derived from fat can have an astounding impact on heart disease by either stalling or reversing it. Numerous studies agree. I firmly believe in these programs, which, please note, also include regular exercise and stress management techniques, but I feel they should only be applied to this specific population.

Eating 10 percent of calories from fat is very difficult to maintain on a long-term basis. It completely eliminates a vast amount of food. For the general population, I believe 20 percent calories from fat is a more realistic goal. Of these 20 percent fat calories, I do not differentiate between saturated fat, polyunsaturated fat, and monounsaturated fat. I agreed with the Food and Drug Administration and the majority of the medical community that saturated fat should be sparingly consumed, especially if an individual has a history of high cholesterol and heart disease. But, and I stress this point, published research findings in the *American Journal of Cardiology* and the *Journal of the American Medical Association,* have shown that the Ornish plan can, in some cases, eliminate the need for surgery. You decide. Say you have been diagnosed with heart disease. You have a clear choice. Would you rather have your chest sawed open, your heart removed, veins grafted from one part of your body and reattached to your heart, the pain, the time, the rehabilitation, the risk of death, the money lost, and the likelihood of it all happening again, or would you rather get with the Ornish or Pritikin programs? Your health insurance will probably pay for the Ornish/Pritikin option because of the overwhelming success rate. Over 150 medical insurance companies accept the Ornish plan alone. That is how enthusiastically insurance companies feel about the plan, and, in my opinion, the only other thing insurance companies get enthusiastic about is raising premiums!

Any program that does not promote exercise is a waste. Study after study conclusively demonstrates that exercise is essential to weight loss and, more important, weight maintenance. If you attempt to lose weight by restricting calories without exercising, your body responds as if you were being starved and consequently burns fewer calories. Exercise must be employed to stimulate the body's metabolic rate and continue the burning of calories at the prediet rate. Thus, you must exercise to lose weight. This is not an option. As you will see with *The Business Plan for the Body,* I don't just talk about exercise, I talk about your *exercise prescription.* You must incorporate cardiovascular exercise, and even more important, strength and resistance training in order to succeed at weight loss. It is not an option.

Let me repeat this point. Your body is smart. Your body wants to stay alive. Your body stores energy, or fat, when you eat more than you expend and utilizes the stored energy—your personal supply of body fat—when you eat fewer calories than your body needs. Your body's metabolism will slow down when you consistently take in less calories than it needs when you are on a diet. The body does not instinctively know that you are overweight, nor would the body ever *want* to be overweight. So when you restrict calories on a diet, the body will slow down to keep you alive longer, even when you have a large supply of

The Business Plan for the Body

fat. That is the body's natural defense. *The only way to combat this phenomenon is to exercise.*

And let me add, the government is now testing two types of diets, a high-protein, low-carbohydrate diet versus the ultra-low-fat, virtually vegetarian diet similar to Dean Ornish's plan. How ridiculous that our government is spending money to test these two programs when every other bit of research indicates that any weight-loss program that does not include exercise is a waste of time and doomed to fail over the long term.

Any weight-loss program that includes the word "quick" is suspect. In Chapter 8 we will look at setting realistic goals and how you can go about achieving them. You will learn that 3,500 calories equals a pound. It is virtually impossible to lose weight quickly and have it be real weight instead of water weight. When I am at the supermarket checkout aisle and I see a magazine cover stating "Lose 5 Pounds in 5 Days," I need to be restrained. Weight gain was not quick, so don't buy into anything that claims to achieve quick weight loss. Most programs that attempt quick weight loss actually achieve nothing but the following: first, they ruin your metabolism by burning lean muscle tissue, which is the most important tissue to preserve; second, they play havoc with your body's water weight. More on this subject in Chapter 8.

3,500 CALORIES EQUALS A POUND

Fasting is yet another option some people opt to employ. I personally fasted every Monday for a number of years. I used it as a way to start the week out "right." Unfortunately, on the Sunday prior and the Tuesday after, I ate like crazy, first in anticipation of the fast and then afterward when I was starving. I know people who fast in order to cleanse toxins from their system. Is it really necessary? The human body has its own built-in detoxification system because the body has its own way of "detoxing" on a regular basis. Your liver, your kidneys, and your intestines filter blood and extract waste products which you naturally eliminate through urine, feces, and even sweat. For the average person, fasting or cleansing is not necessary.

Fasting is problematic as it drastically lowers an individual's basal metabolic rate. About a day's worth of carbohydrates are stored in your liver and muscles. Once that is depleted, you begin to burn not just body fat but muscle as well. And, let's face it, who can keep up a fast, or would want to, for a long period of time? Long-term fasting can seriously damage vital physiological processes, given that it eliminates the necessary vitamins and minerals to survive. So unless you are Dick Gregory, Mahatma Gandhi, or some other individual with a political cause to publicize—forget the fasting.

Your preconceived notions need to be explored as potential competition in the weight-loss business. You need to examine your beliefs about fitness and weight loss, because they may shed a great deal of light on your current situation. *Your beliefs, if they are incorrect, may be the single greatest competitive barrier to your success.* These beliefs exist within you, either consciously or subconsciously, so you have to be honest with yourself and examine them. I have heard each and every one of these fallacies hundreds, possibly thousands, of times over the years from clients, family members, friends, acquaintances, competitors, and the media. Trust me, they are all false. Some of these fallacies are explored below. For others, which will require more detail, I will direct you to the appropriate chapter that covers that topic in greater depth.

*F*allacy 1: I have a bad metabolism.

This is the most frequently mentioned fallacy I hear from overweight individuals. In Chapter 5, "The Financials," we are going to do a complete analysis of metabolism and its components, which include lean muscle tissue, physical activity, digestion, and more. If you need to skip to that chapter right now to get answers to your questions regarding metabolism, do so. I would bet big money that your metabolism is just fine, it is your *behavior* that is not. The Obesity Research Center in New York City conducted a study to examine the behavior of obese individuals who claimed they could not lose weight through dieting. All individuals attributed their inability to shed pounds to their slow metabolism. Guess what? The researchers found that most of the obese participants were grossly underestimating the calories they consumed by more than half. It was not their metabolism that caused them to be overweight, it was their high consumption of calories.

STOP BLAMING YOUR METABOLISM

Fallacy 2: I have bad genes.

In Chapter 5 we also discuss the role of genes. John Foreyt, Ph.D., an obesity expert at Baylor College of Medicine's Nutrition Research Clinic in Houston, says that on average, one-quarter of a person's weight may be determined by genetics. That means three-quarters is environmental and within your control. Furthermore, consider the fact that a genetic predisposition is vastly different from a predetermined one. Most overweight parents raise overweight children by teaching them how to overeat and by not encouraging activity. So yes, a portion of your metabolism is dictated by genes. Two people, same age, height, weight, etc., who begin my plan, will lose weight at different speeds because of the genetic component involved. But bottom line, they *both will lose weight.* Repeating, *they both will lose weight.*

Look at the difference between Americans and Europeans. Michael Fumento, author of *The Fat of the Land: The Obesity Epidemic and How Overweight Americans Can Help Themselves,* notes that Americans are a full sixteen pounds heavier than their cousins in western Europe. We know that as a nation, the number of obese Americans has doubled in the past ten years. Is it possible for our genetic makeup to have changed so drastically in that brief period of time? It would seem unlikely.

Take the whole genetic argument one step further. Say one person tests better than another. The better tester may have a better memory. Is memory influenced by genes? Probably. Does this mean "bad testers" should quit school because of their impaired memory, or should they realize that they need to work harder than their friends to achieve good grades, or employ a different studying strategy? The same applies to sports. Do you tell your son or daughter, who does not appear to have innate physical ability, to just give it up and not exercise or participate in any sports? That would be like saying, "You don't run very well so forget sports." I hope the parent would say, "You go out there and give it your all. If your friend is a faster runner, so be it. Maybe you hit the ball harder or make more baskets. And it doesn't matter if you don't. The point is to enjoy the game and the activity." I'm not

IT'S YOUR BEHAVIOR, NOT YOUR GENES

your parent, but I can be your cheerleader. You go out there and conquer weight loss. I don't care about your genes, I care about your behavior. You can do it. You can be in the weight-loss business.

Everything about us has a genetic component. But there is a *behavioral* component as well. Yes, for the last time, if one hundred thousand million zillion people go on my plan to lose weight, they each will lose weight at a different pace, but—and remember this every time someone gives you the genes argument—*each and every person will ultimately lose weight.*

*F*allacy 3: I have a thyroid problem.

I know I am sounding like a broken record, but once again, Chapter 5 (maybe you should just flip to it now and read it) will cover all your questions regarding thyroid and its role in the body. According to researchers at Johns Hopkins University, underactive thyroid problems are present in about eleven million Americans, or 4 percent of the population, mostly women and the elderly. Yet, as we have established, approximately 20 percent of Americans are obese, or 20 percent heavier than their ideal body weight. And 50.7 percent of women and 59.4 percent of men are overweight. If you think you have thyroid dysfunction, go get a blood test and obtain the data. Johns Hopkins University researchers advise adults thirty-five and older to have what is called a sensitive TSH (thyroid stimulating hormone) test every five years. This simple blood test, which will cost about fifty dollars, detects thyroid disease in its earliest stages. Odds are overwhelming that you don't have a thyroid problem, but Chapter 5 will give you the information you need to determine if you do.

*F*allacy 4: I am eating fat-free or low-fat.

The creation of so-called fat-free and low-fat foods, and the belief that fat-free equates to calorie-free, is one of the principal reasons that the American population has virtually ballooned in girth. Keep in mind, almost every food has fat. Yes, even fruits and vegetables can have a small percentage of fat. I do not believe that fat alone is the culprit, though high consumption of fat in our diets is unhealthy, especially saturated fat, otherwise known as the "bad" fat. Fat is actually necessary in our diet. Seizing upon the fact that fat is the enemy, food manufacturers identified a terrific consumer market niche over the last ten years by producing, marketing, and labeling foods as "fat-free" or "low-fat" or "light." Even foods such as jelly, jam, pasta, bagels, bread, and angel food cake, which always had very little to no fat, suddenly began splashing across their labels the words "fat-free." The American populace totally embraced the concept of fat-free, equating it to calorie-free, and went on a binge.

But isn't the fat-free or low-fat version of a product lower in calories than the real thing? Good question. The answer, sometimes yes, sometimes no. It depends on the product, and keep in mind—as we established in our discussion of programs that claim sugar is the culprit—most manufacturers took the fat out and replaced it with added sugar and, in most cases, sodium. Cookies, salad dressing, and ice cream are just a few of the many items that have experienced this trend. Observe the following chart:

FAT-FREE IS NOT CALORIE-FREE

ORIGINAL VERSUS LIGHT AND FAT-FREE VERSION

REAL THING	LIGHT VERSION	FAT-FREE VERSION
Pepperidge Farm Double Chocolate Milano Cookie 140 calories for 2 cookies 8 grams of fat	SnackWell's Creme Sandwich Cookie 110 calories for 2 cookies 3 grams of fat	Archway Fat-Free Devil's Food Cookie 140 calories for 2 cookies 0 grams of fat
Newman's Own Ranch Dressing 140 calories for 2 tablespoons 15 grams of fat	Hidden Valley Light Ranch Dressing 80 calories for 2 tablespoons 7 grams of fat	Kraft Fat-Free Ranch Dressing 50 calories for 2 tablespoons 0 grams of fat
Häagen Dazs Pistachio Ice Cream 290 for half cup 20 grams of fat	Ben & Jerry's Low-Fat Cherry Garcia 170 for half cup 3 grams of fat	Edy's Fat-Free Cookie Yogurt 110 for half cup 0 grams of fat

As you can see, Milano cookies are only 30 calories more per serving than SnackWell's, but the same amount of calories per serving as the Archway fat-free. You probably thought there would be a greater disparity. If you were only going to eat two cookies, then in my opinion it doesn't make an appreciable difference. But do not, I repeat, do not think that light or fat-free cookies are much fewer in calories than the real thing. They aren't.

With regards to salad dressing, Newman's Own Ranch Dressing has almost three times as many calories as the fat-free variety. The Hidden Valley Light Ranch is 80 calories for two tablespoons, but dressings such as Ranch, Thousand Island, and French tend to be dense, which means they do not spread throughout the salad. This promotes you to use more. In general, Americans put far too much dressing on salads, especially when it is fat-free. Once again they equate fat-free to calorie-free. Use salad dressing sparingly, put it on the side or be smart and try balsamic vinegar or lemon, both of which are tasty and very low in calories.

As is obvious from the ice cream/frozen yogurt illustration on our chart, the heavy-creamed Häagen Dazs is almost triple the calories of the Edy's Fat-Free Cookie Yogurt. The Ben & Jerry's is lower in calories than the Häagen Dazs, but still contains 170 calories for only one-half of a cup. I would wager the average serving of ice cream/frozen yogurt is more in the range of two or more cups, four times the serving size listed. For the Edy's Fat-Free Cookie Yogurt, that would equate to 440 calories. We won't even discuss the thought of two cups of Häagen Dazs (which, by the way, is the entire pint), which would total 1,160 calories!

Important point. According to the USDA, in order to use the term "light" on a label, a product must contain one-third fewer calories than the original *or* half the fat of the original. Notice the use of the word "or." So it is legal for a product to use the term "light" in its name, yet the product could have the same amount of calories as the original. Terminology such as this can be misleading to individuals, which underscores the need to read labels carefully.

CREATE A CALORIC DEFICIT

As you will learn in subsequent chapters, every calorie counts. Losing weight is all about creating a caloric deficit. You will learn to count calories because caloric intake determines weight loss or weight gain. My recommendation is to keep fat intake—whether it be saturated, polyunsaturated, or monounsaturated fat—down to around 20 percent of your daily caloric intake. But if you do go over in the percent-

The Business Plan for the Body

age of fat, but stay within your target of total calories consumed to lose weight, I say fine, unless you have other issues at hand, such as high cholesterol, heart disease, high blood pressure, cancer, or some other condition that requires you to be more rigid with regard to fat (especially saturated fat) intake. Repeat with me,

"It's not the fat, it's the calories."

*F*allacy 5: I just can't lose weight.

On a nationally syndicated talk show, a woman appeared who had forty-five pounds of fat removed by liposuction. She beamed as she sat down and said, "Diet, exercise, and weight-loss programs didn't work for me. My body just couldn't lose weight." Wrong. I promise you she has never really been on a program, and the doctor who removed forty-five pounds of fat was giving her a quick fix, and at great risk. There is a risk of death with liposuction. According to a survey of board-certified plastic surgeons between 1994 and 1998, the mortality rate was 19.1 deaths per 100,000 liposuction procedures. That translates to about one death per five thousand liposuction procedures. That's right, there is an actual possibility you can die on the operating table having liposuction. That may not seem like a high percentage, but it will to you, your family, and friends if you happen to be that one out of five thousand. The entire weight-loss industry is loaded with people trying to sell you a quick fix, but I know you realize that a fast fix just doesn't get the job done!

I came across an Ann Landers column featuring a letter from a fifty-six-year-old woman complaining about the lack of large-size clothing for women. She claimed that diets didn't work for her and neither did exercise. Her weight, just for the record, was 270 pounds. Does this sound as ludicrous to you as it does to me? Do you realize that this woman must consume thousands of calories a day in order to keep her weight at 270 pounds? I bet exercise is not working for her because she *isn't* doing any.

YES, YOU *CAN* LOSE WEIGHT

The Competition

Here is another thought. Your plane goes down, you land on a deserted island, there is a severely limited supply of food. Three months later you are rescued and come staggering out of the forest. What's the visual? The rescuers encounter a plump survivor who, when queried as to his well-fed appearance states, "I just can't lose weight." That is certainly not the survivor picture I remember seeing over the years.

Yes, you can lose weight, but a common problem I do see is that most diets are so drastic that a person cannot adhere to them for more than a couple of days. I blame the media.

YOU CAN'T LOSE TEN POUNDS IN TEN DAYS

How many programs make ridiculous claims like "Lose Ten Pounds in Ten Days"? Let's get serious, to lose ten pounds in ten days you would have to exercise enough to burn 35,000 calories more than you consumed, which would probably require you to trek the Himalayas ten hours a day for ten days or be locked in a closet without food. We are going to address the reality of weight loss in Chapter 8, but for now, realize that any program you go on is for life, not for a brief period of time.

I also frequently overhear people complain, as they are exercising, that they can't lose weight. Yes they can, but they are in the "I exercise so I can eat what I want" syndrome. This is very common. I see people killing themselves working out only to eat back the calories they just burned a few minutes ago. I had a former employee who used to say to his clients when he left each session, "Don't undo all the good work you just did." Basically he was politely saying, "Stop overeating!"

In my opinion, if you are exercising consistently and not losing weight, then you're either exercising improperly or, more likely, overeating. Overexercising will only lead to an overuse injury. How? Well, you eat, eat, eat, then you exercise, exercise, exercise to burn off the additional calories consumed. In a matter of time your back, knees, neck, or feet are bound to give out from the excessive exercise. Don't do it. Exercise intelligently and count your calories. That is the key to weight loss.

Any person can lose weight. Repeat, any person can lose weight. You just have to be intelligent, honest with yourself, patient, and on plan! Remember, it took you months, if not years, to gain the weight. It will take time to lose that weight.

Fallacy 6: I'm fat but fit.

This is a fallacy that has recently been added to my list. You simply cannot be fat and fit. What many people may mean by this is that through cardiovascular conditioning they are in better shape than if they were not exercising. Cardiovascular exercise improves an individual's ability to supply blood to working muscles. As cardiovascular functions improve, an overweight individual can climb stairs easier, play tennis, walk on a treadmill, or take aerobic classes. I think that's great, but you still have to make weight loss your primary goal to save your body on a long-term basis.

Being overweight means that your risk of serious illness such as heart disease, stroke, cancer, and diabetes is increased. If you are overweight, you are requiring your heart to work overtime to supply blood to all the additional body fat, you are requiring your stomach to work overtime to digest the additional food, you are requiring your pancreas to secrete additional insulin, and so on. The bottom line: You are overworking your internal organs. This overuse does not make one fit.

BEING FAT IS NOT BEING FIT

You are also overworking your joints. I promise you, after repeated impact, the knee joints, lower back, and feet will begin to present problems when additional weight is present. Doesn't it seem like the whole world is getting knee surgery? In my thirteen-year experience, almost everyone I know who is overweight and exercising will eventually experience pain and discomfort, which will probably lead to surgery or physical therapy and ultimately bring their program to a halt.

Look at it this way. Yes, you can be relatively healthy for a fat person, just as you can be relatively healthy for somebody with AIDS. But obesity attacks your body in a myriad of ways.

Are you going into the "weight loss" business or the "I'm overweight but fit" business? I would hope it would be the former rather than the latter.

Fallacy 7: My body has plateaued.

Let me be as succinct as possible on this issue: Your body has not plateaued, *your program has.* Here is one of my favorite fitness expressions:

What does this mean? Simple, you must confuse your body in order to force it to change.

A former neighbor started a walking program. I saw her in her walking clothes and did what I always do when I see someone attempting an exercise program. I praised her. Approximately one month later I asked her how she was doing. She said, "Great. I've lost four pounds!" I told her how proud I was of her and wished her continued success. Two months went by and I never saw her in exercise clothing. Finally I asked her, "So, how is your walking program?" She said, "Oh, I quit that last month. My body plateaued and I stopped losing weight."

Wrong, wrong, wrong. Her body did not plateau, her program did. We are going to talk about the exercise prescription, and the progression of that prescription, in Chapters 7 and 9, but for now let's just say my neighbor's body was changing from the walking but then it adapted. I always say that your body is very, very intelligent. It will change for you as long as you keep challenging it. Once the challenge is over, so is the change. Once again, if you only put your body through the same old paces, it no longer has to work as hard, which translates into burning fewer calories. Your program has reached a plateau.

WITHOUT CHALLENGE, THERE IS NO CHANGE

*F*allacy 8: My body wants to be this weight.

Marilyn Wann, a San Francisco leader of the National Association to Advance Fat Acceptance and the author of *Fat! So?*, claims her 270 pounds on a five-foot-four frame was her natural size. I think this is absolutely ridiculous. Bodies want to be overweight and out of shape? They want to be? This is totally untrue. Think about it for a moment. Say you are a women, five feet five inches tall, who for forty-eight years weighed between 120 and 125 pounds. All of a sudden you are struggling to keep your weight under 150 pounds and would be thrilled to weigh 145 pounds consistently. What happened? Yes, with menopause many women have to work harder than ever to keep their weight under control because, at the onset of menopause, a woman goes from losing seven-tenths of a pound of muscle a year to losing one full pound each year. As we will learn, this will clearly cause a woman's basal metabolic rate to decline, but it can be reversed through strength and resistance exercise.

I have overheard numerous people over the years, just like Ms. Wann, say, "My body is just comfortable at this weight," or "It just wants to be this weight." On the contrary, because of the tremendous stresses placed on your internal organs as well as your muscles and joints by additional pounds, your body is uncomfortable at a high weight. We will learn in Chapter 5 that metabolically, the body speeds up when we overeat, in an attempt to shed the added calories. Why, then, could any intelligent person say that "my body just wants to be this weight"?

YOUR BODY DOES NOT WANT TO BE OVERWEIGHT

As the body ages, the risk factors for certain illnesses increase. Furthermore, these risks are exacerbated with added weight, so in essence you are increasing your risk. As we age, what better time to get in the best shape possible? That can be achieved by keeping body weight in check and not allowing it to rise to its so-called natural size.

Or think about it this way. You buy a brand-new car and maintain it properly, regular oil and filter changes, frequent checkups, wash and wax. The car looks and performs great. Then it gets a little older, you get sloppy with the routine maintenance, you don't fix the dents, you let the car go. Before you know it, your vehicle looks terrible and runs even worse. What if you had taken better care of the car as it aged? What if you made a point to keep it in tip-top shape, inside and out, as it got older? I know you would like the car more, enjoy driving it, take greater pride in owning it, save yourself money and make owning this vehicle a winning experience. Then again, just junk it and buy a new one, as most Americans do when the wear and tear begins to occur.

MAKE REPAIRS, YOU CAN'T JUNK YOUR BODY

Now think about your body. You can't junk it as it ages. You can't trade it in. This is your one and only body. Do you really want to be heavy and possess an out-of-shape body? Can't you start doing repairs, right now, and alter your body's current decline? Again, the choice is yours. Do the maintenance. Just don't try to convince me that your body wants to be over-weight. What your body wants is a winning experience.

*F*allacy 9: *I'm young, I can do what I want.*

Here is a shocking statistic. A study from the National Institutes of Health confirms that in 1985–86 the average weight for Americans was 161 pounds for the twenty-five to thirty-year-old age group. In 1992–93 that number went up a full ten pounds. This is a disaster, and we're not even discussing children, whose weight has also increased dramatically during this time period. I deal with many people in their forties through nineties. During each initial consultation, I always ask a person's weight when they were twenty, thirty, forty, fifty, and so on. Frequently, these people never experienced weight gain until their latter thirties to forties. Now, research shows that individuals in their mid- to late twenties are up ten pounds in weight. What will happen in their thirties and forties? More and more weight gain. You cannot overeat and underexercise no matter what your age. Remember my car analogy: Buy a new car and abuse the hell out of it, how long will that car look and act new? Don't change the oil, beat up the transmission, forgo wash and wax, and delay servicing the vehicle, and I promise you in no time you will possess an old-looking, poorly performing automobile. Same applies to your body. Take care of it now, maintain it, and it will give you a long-term healthy run. Don't gain weight in your twenties. Don't gain weight ever. If you have gained weight, get it together now and don't let a ten-pound problem become a twenty-, thirty-, forty-, or fifty-pound disaster in the future. This is just like debt. Overspend a little bit, pay it off over the next few months. Overspend a lot, and it will take you years to pay it off.

*F*allacy 10: *I'm big-boned.*

I started my fitness career as an aerobics instructor. I used to teach huge classes at two of Chicago's most popular clubs. One frequent student was a young woman you would refer to as "muscular," "firm," "athletic," "big-boned," and all those other politically correct terms used to substitute for the obvious—fat. About three years after I ceased teaching and devoted myself to full-time personal training, I was lifting weights in a gym, and in walks the former stu-

NO, YOU DON'T HAVE BIG BONES

dent with this magnificent, lean, long body. She looked like a ballet dancer. I walked up to her and said, "You look great. You have lost so much weight." She remembered me and we proceeded to chat. She had adjusted her program to include strength and resistance training, pulled back on the cardio, and paid attention to her eating.

Before our conversation ended, I just couldn't resist asking her this question. I said, "Please don't take offense, but did everyone used to tell you that you were 'big-boned'?" She laughed and said yes. She then proceeded to lift up her sparrowlike wrist and say, "Do these look big to you? I was fat, not big-boned, and once the weight came off I finally saw my true size."

You are not big-boned. Yes, some of you may possess a wider, taller, or longer frame, but, bottom line, the skeletal size of the average man and woman does not vary that much. Go to your nearest natural history museum. Do you notice a great difference in the bone size of the skeletons on display? No. Then stop believing that you are big-boned. Your weight is the issue, not your bone size.

Fallacy 11: I'm too muscular.

This fallacy is popular with women since few men would use the excuse that they are "too muscular." Women who are overweight frequently tell me that they are too muscular. You will learn (Chapter 5) that after the age of twenty, the average person loses seven-tenths of a pound of muscle each year. You will also learn that an individual can only regain or rebuild muscle through strength and resistance training. How is it then that a fifty-five-year-old woman, five feet four inches tall, 175 pounds, can claim to be too muscular, when she hasn't exercised in years? She can't be too muscular. What she is is overweight. Now she may not jiggle, or have cellulite, which we often equate with being overweight, but trust me, her added weight is not muscle. It is marbleized fat, just like a good piece of prime beef filet. Genetically, some women appear firmer and more solid than others, but that does not mean they are any less fat than someone with no muscle tone. Recall what I just said about being "big-boned"?

I have been aggressively performing strength and resistance training four to five times a week for almost two decades. I work very hard to maintain, and increase, my lean muscle tissue.

There is no way that a woman who "flirts" with weight training is going to become too muscular.

You will learn in Chapter 5 that muscle is the body's most metabolically active tissue. It burns lots of calories around the clock. So if you believe you're muscular, then you're presently burning many calories a day. So how can you be overweight? There is no logic to this argument. Sorry.

Fallacy 12: I don't eat.

I have to use a personal experience to approach this subject. My grandmother, Yia Yia in Greek, died a few years ago at the age of eighty-five. She was five-foot-four and probably born at 160 pounds because, prior to dying of colon cancer, that was her lifelong weight. As she had high blood pressure and some other health concerns, I would ask her, delicately, "Yia Yia, don't you think it would help you if you lost a few pounds?" She would reply, "How could I lose weight? As it is, I never eat." Well, I was fortunate enough to be in Greece with her at one point and personally witness what she referred to as "never eating." If "never eating" meant standing at the stove, cooking and tasting everything that came in and out of the kitchen, then I guess one could call that "never eating." I watched Yia Yia eating around the clock, but never sitting down, as did her younger sister. Her "never eating" should have been called "never eating at the table." Evidently, she believed that calories consumed in a standing mode do not count.

IF YOU'RE OVERWEIGHT, YOU OVEREAT

Similar to "never eating," here is another favorite: "I eat like a bird." This is the first excuse I totally agree with. You probably do eat like a bird. Birds eat a *tremendous* amount of food. How do you think they have the energy to fly all day? Are you active and flying in the air hour upon hour every day?

If you are overweight, you do eat. You overeat. We already heard the research that most people underestimate their caloric intake by one-half. Escalation in body weight is due to overeating. So trust me, you do eat, a lot! Perhaps you are not aware of it, but nonetheless, it is occurring.

Fallacy 13: The scale doesn't matter.

This aversion to the scale is possibly at the heart of your problem. The only way to get the truth about whether you are

The Business Plan for the Body

on or off plan is to get on the scale, which we will explore in more detail in Chapter 8. You must know the facts. The scale is your best friend on a weight-loss program because it doesn't lie. You must weigh yourself once a week, at the same time of the day, in order to assess your progress.

Just a note, please don't get on the scale five times a day. I have had numerous clients over the years who call me at seven A.M. and say, "I am so happy with your program, I lost 1.5 pounds," only to call back at ten A.M. and say, "Well, I knew it was only short-lived, now I am only down one pound," etc., throughout the day. This is crazy. Your body weight will fluctuate according to what you have to eat and drink. So weigh yourself once a week, same time, same place, and let that be your guide.

NUMBERS DO MATTER

One more point. If you haven't been on the scale for a long time, and for some of you that may be years, don't be surprised when you weigh more than you thought.

I equate overeating with overspending. If you never check your bank balance, you will have no idea how much money is in your account. But once you are out of money, the bank is kind enough to bounce your checks as a way of saying, "You are overspending and I am not going to pay for it." Wouldn't it be wonderful if the same thing were to happen with your eating? You would bring the fork up to your mouth filled with pecan pie à la mode and a hand would come out, grab the fork, and a voice would state, "Hey, who do you think you are, eating this bite? You are way over today's caloric allocation (more on this in Chapter 6). Put the fork down! Go work out!" That could save your life, and probably thousands of others a year.

Fallacy 14: I diet five days out of every week and never lose weight.

If I am interpreting this statement correctly, you are saying that you diet Monday through Friday of every week, but then eat whatever you want on the weekends, and never lose weight. I totally agree. Do you know why you never lose weight? There is a very simple explanation. As you will learn in the following chapters, weight loss is achieved by creating a caloric deficit. Basically, you have to expend more calories than

DON'T DIET PART-TIME

you consume to lose weight. If, from Monday through Friday, you create a caloric deficit, you are on your way to losing weight. But if you then follow those five days of undereating with two days of overeating, odds are you will never lose weight. You're lucky you're not gaining weight. Why?

For the sake of example, let's say that for five consecutive days you create a caloric deficit of 500 calories a day. After five days you are down 2,500 calories. If on Saturday and Sunday you overeat, you will take in those 2,500 calories and possibly more. Here is how it works. Saturday morning you "treat" yourself to a Denver omelette, about 800 calories. You have some pizza at lunch and a salad with lots of dressing, another 1,000 calories. Then some chips in front of the television, 500 additional calories, topped off with dinner out, maybe pasta with Alfredo sauce, a steak, fried potatoes, dessert, etc. Am I making my point? There is no way you can diet for five days, then undo all that hard work in two days, and ever expect to lose weight.

Think of it this way: You save money 364 days out of the year. Then on the 365th day, you blow that money. The next day you're back to square one. Savings gone, money spent. Same applies to weight loss. There is no such thing as a "part-time" plan. You are either on plan or off. Remember my discussion of the light switch in Chapter 1, "The Mission Statement." You are either on or off program. If the switch is "on" you are fully committed to the plan. If you think you are going to succeed with a five-day-a-week program, you are mistaken. Full compliance—that is the road to success.

*F*allacy 15: I am having a bad day so what the hell.

Eating one generous piece of cake is probably adding 500 calories to your daily caloric intake. But if you have the cake, then decide you've blown it and have two pieces of Godiva chocolate, followed by a cappuccino, a few biscotti, and half a piece of cheesecake, you just added 1,000 calories to the 500 additional you already ate. You're up 1,500 calories instead of 500. Your body does not say, "Oh, Judy is having a bad day since she already blew her diet. Today she can eat whatever she wants. Tomorrow she will go back on plan." No matter what your mind is saying, the body registers every calorie you take in. If you overeat, whether it's

YOUR BODY
REGISTERS
EVERY CALORIE
YOU EAT

The Business Plan for the Body

because of a birthday or a bad day, your body will register each and every calorie you eat. You can easily turn a treat into a disaster. One splurge may take you a few days to burn off, another may take you a few weeks. And for the shorter people out there, you will find that it is harder for you to create a caloric deficit than it is for taller individuals. Depending on your eating patterns and activity level, a big splurge could take you a solid two weeks to burn off.

Look at it another way. Back to my spending analogy. If you save your money all month, then go out and splurge on, say, a cashmere sweater or a tennis racket, you treated yourself and called it a day. But what if you follow that splurge with ten more things that are in the "splurge" category. You went overboard. You probably put them on your credit card and really made a mess of things. It may take you months, even years, to pay off this overindulgence. Before the days of plastic, you had to save the money in advance in order to spend the money. Now the reverse is the case. Prior to the industrial revolution, food was not as available and plentiful. Sweets and fatty meats were served only on special occasions. Now, for most Americans, every day is a special occasion. You have to go back to "the numbers." You simply cannot say that today is a "bad" day so just eat whatever you want. If you believe I am wrong, then you don't believe in the power of the calorie. The "bad" days will stay with your body for days, weeks, perhaps even years to come.

Be realistic. If you had more food at lunch than you anticipated in your plan, then scale back at dinner. Similarly, if you went with your spouse for a special anniversary dinner, cut back the next few days and get rid of the unwanted calories. Remember, your body doesn't want those additional calories and will thank you for getting rid of them as soon as possible. Get on the scale the next day. Get the data, then crunch the numbers.

Fallacy 16: "It's either the face or the hips."

I remember a few years ago when a famous actress who'd gained weight said in an interview that as a woman ages, she has to increase her weight because it is either "the face or the hips." I believe she meant that as a woman ages her face will become thin and wrinkled, a transformation that can be reversed by gaining weight. Therefore, to maintain a full face, she has to live with larger hips. This is absolutely nutty. A woman can have a healthy, full face *and* lean hips. She simply has to embrace one simple fact—she must exercise.

I am certain that there are additional fallacies I am omitting, but these are the most common. Think a moment. Do you have a belief that is keeping you from succeeding? Do you believe you can lose weight? Do you really have a bad metabolism, genes, or a thyroid problem? Has eating fat-free worked? Go back to your mission statement, which I will ask you to do numerous times, and decide: Do you want to be in the weight-loss business? If the desire is not there, I can pretty much guarantee you won't be a success. If the desire is there, stay with me for the next important step.

STRATEGIC ACTION PLAN

You're launching a business, the weight-loss business. Obviously, you do not want to fail in this endeavor, so you examine the competitive strategies that exist in the marketplace. You quickly determine that these competitive plans, even those that do temporarily achieve some measure of success, all possess significant negative side effects; they are all flawed.

You have additionally reviewed any preconceived thoughts you possess regarding weight loss and how they relate to you. And most important, you've discarded those thoughts that you now realize no longer realistically apply.

You once again recall your mission statement: You are in the weight-loss business and your "profit" is weight loss. You currently have in your hands the guide that will enable your business plan to succeed, *The Business Plan for the Body*. Read it from cover to cover. Stay up all night if you need to, just read it. And by all means, eat all the broccoli you desire while you study a business strategy that will create a business winner—you.

Like Thomas Edison, you may have found ten thousand ways that didn't work, but also just like Tom, you've now discovered one that does. It's time to flip that switch to on!

GOING PUBLIC

3 *Your IPO: Getting the Word Out*

A young woman in her early thirties used to spend $10,000 to $12,000 a year training with my firm. She holds both a law and MBA degree and is employed by a Fortune 500 company. She is extremely overweight. She virtually lives on cereal, pastry, doughnuts, ribs, fast food from McDonald's, Taco Bell, etc. She claims that even the thought of fresh fruit could make her vomit. Each week she called my office to complain about her lack of weight loss. Each time I asked, "How did you do with your eating last night?" She replied, "Oh, I ate everything because people would notice if I were picking at my food." My response, "Well, don't they know that you're trying to lose weight?" "Oh no," she replied, "no one knows." When I asked why, she said, "They would all be disappointed in me if I failed." So she refuses to tell anyone that she is trying to lose weight, from her friends to her coworkers to her family. Why, you might ask? What is the real reason? The reason is simple: She planned to fail. She is not thinking about other people and their reaction, she is thinking about herself. She planned to fail, and made every effort to be successful in her failure quest.

That's right, most people start a weight-loss program planning to fail. Pressure and support can help you stay on plan.

> **"We are not interested in the possibilities of defeat."**
> **QUEEN VICTORIA**

Let's take a moment to look at where we are. First, remember the mission statement: weight loss. Second, we looked at the competition's strategy and determined that our plan will be infinitely better and will yield significant longer lasting results with no negative side effects. We examined all the excuses and preconceived notions we have relied on in the past that have prevented us from focusing on our "plan" and sabotaged our success. Now it's time to *go public*.

Most people start a weight-loss program consciously or subconsciously planning to fail, privately. Most business organizations, just like you, began their operation in private, though certainly not with the idea they would fail. They started their "lives" as privately held entities created by a single entrepreneur or group of entrepreneurs. As a privately held organization, all information regarding the inner workings of the company remained behind "closed doors." Revenues, expenses, management compensation, etc., were known only to the business owner and perhaps a small group of the senior management team. The outside business community knew very little regarding the inner workings or financials of the organization. The company may appear successful, perhaps even unsuccessful, yet the investment community can only conjecture. That's the luxury of being private; no external pressure, no public knowledge, no shame. The same applies to you. If you haven't screamed to the world that you are in the weight-loss business, and you don't lose weight—well, no one will know that you tried and failed. But you know what? You'll know.

PLAN NOT TO FAIL

Once a business organization has a proven track record of revenue growth, earnings, and market share, it may decide that in order to grow, it will need to raise capital. One way to raise capital comes through a share offering usually referred to as an IPO (initial public offering). Once a company decides it is necessary to go public, an entirely new environment is created. The same applies to you going public. You, too, will operate in a new environment. The business organization must file the appropriate documents with the Securities and Exchange Commission; senior management travels the country conducting "road shows" for potential investors, explaining the ins and outs of the company—the financials, the management team, their compensation, basically everything is now made public. In essence, management is presenting its plan to the public. In the future, earning estimates will be disclosed, so if they aren't achieved, investors will know. The investors who purchase shares in the new public company now have a financial stake in the company's future and will apply pressure on management to achieve the goals it has stated. That's what we want for you. Just like the newly public organization, we want you to be out there stating your goals and explaining your business plan. And keep in mind, at least you don't have to scream yours in magazines, newspapers, on television, over the Internet, and then have financial analysts poring over your results.

Why am I telling you to "go public" before you have achieved a weight-loss success? Simple. By announcing your goals to those with whom you come in regular contact, you will be educating your "management team" and others around you to understand your new business venture: weight loss.

ANNOUNCE YOUR INTENT

You want everyone to clearly understand your mission statement. If they don't, they will assume you are still in the weight-gain business, as you have appeared to be in the past. Share with them your mission statement: "I am going into the weight-loss business. I am going to succeed at losing weight." You need to do your own personal "dog and pony show." As I just said, companies going public frequently travel around the country, possibly the world, presenting to potential investors and analysts their mission statement and their strategy for achieving success with that mission. The same applies to you. You're about to conduct your own public road show.

Start with your significant other. If you don't have one, then your best friend. Sit him or her down, preferably not over a cheesecake, and clearly state your mission statement. From there go down the line of friends, business associates, family, and anyone else you come in contact with on a regular basis. Tell them.

Over the years, I am often so disappointed when people say to me at the initial consultation, "Please don't tell the doorman, and I definitely don't want one of your other clients coming up to me at a party and saying, 'Hey, I hear you're working with Jim Karas.'" This is such a mistake. I believe people don't want to go public because they plan to fail. Once again, most people start a weight-loss program planning to fail, and it's much more comfortable to fail privately than publicly.

You may not be aware that your subconscious is planning to fail even though your conscious mind wants to succeed. An individual may consciously want to succeed at weight loss, but subconsciously be afraid of success because he or she will then be evaluated in a different context. An example of this would be an individual who was passed over for a promotion and blamed his or her weight for the oversight. What would happen if that same individual lost weight and still did not get the promotion? He or she would have to examine issues unrelated to their weight, a frightening thought for many. I went over this issue when I asked you if you were ready to go into the weight-loss business. You must explore this often-present psychological component.

As I noted previously, by going public you're putting pressure on yourself to follow through with the plan. Pressure is hard, but check this out. Go up to any successful individual you know and ask one of the following:

- *Was there pressure on you when you were climbing the corporate ladder, or*
- *Was there pressure on you when you started your own business, perhaps had to borrow money from friends, in-laws, or*
- *Was there pressure on you when you were in medical school, graduate school, working part-time to pay for school, or*
- *Was there pressure on you to meet the payroll for your employees?*

Please don't kid yourself that success is achieved without pressure. During the last thirteen years I have been fortunate enough to spend time with some of the most successful men and women in this country. As with any relationship, we began to share stories of our lives. Time after time I would hear stories of incredible hard work and discipline, the "all nighters," the missed vacations, the difficult boss, the juggling of children, the merger, the missed earnings projections, and the lost job. I heard countless stories of pressure, but most of all I heard an overwhelming desire and determination to succeed. Note, these individuals did not quit. On the contrary, they learned from past mistakes, regrouped, and forged ahead. They simply wouldn't stop until they attained their goal. People look at them today and remark, "Oh,

MAKE PRESSURE A POSITIVE FORCE

The Business Plan for the Body

they were so lucky." Nonsense. They made that "luck," they strived for that "luck." It may appear simple, but believe me, it wasn't.

It isn't simple for me. Every day I make it clear to people around me that I am on plan. I talk about it. I realize that this bugs some individuals. I hear the lame attempts at levity, "Here comes the food police, eat up," as I enter a room. I don't care, I like the way I now look and feel. I am on plan.

So often I have people approach me and say, "Don't you want cake, don't you want fries, don't you want really *good* food?" Sure, I like to eat these things, but they will screw up my plan. If I eat food that contains an additional 500 calories, then the next day I have to either put in more time exercising or reduce my caloric intake by 500 calories. I do not want to do either. So I don't eat the food. And to those who view me as a "food Nazi," let me say, "There is an entire food world out there that is tasty, fulfilling, won't throw an individual off of plan, and will keep me in size-thirty-one-waist jeans."

Robert Jeffrey, an epidemiologist at the University of Minnesota, conducted the following case study. First, he recruited 166 adults to follow a program designed to melt excess fat. Half of the volunteers were asked to come alone, while the rest were encouraged to bring three friends. After ten months, those who had joined with a friend fared best. They stuck with the program, had lost about 30 percent more weight, and were more likely to have kept it off than the people who signed up alone. Once again, the more people you get excited and interested in improving their health, weight, and appearance, the more you personally enhance your chances of success.

My firm had an overweight client for years who was a successful real estate developer. She told me that whenever she tried to order salads with dressing on the side and grilled fish with no oil, everyone at the table would roll their eyes as if to say, "Right, and on the way home she'll stop for a cheeseburger, fries, and a shake." I know she's correct. People doubt her commitment to stay on plan, because so many overweight individuals, when they are out and about, are conscious that people are observing their eating and will purposely eat little, and then gorge themselves in private. What my client and others like her should have said is, "Listen, I have struggled with this for a long time, I am going to succeed at weight loss. I have a plan." They undoubtedly would have been more sympathetic and encouraging. Again, it's making one's plan public.

Sometimes an individual goes public in a very unintended manner as in a heart attack or stroke. These do qualify as public events; however, even after such traumas, some blithely continue to systematically annihilate themselves with fatty foods and absolutely no exercise regime. Remember the television sitcom, *Roseanne*? The actor, John Goodman, who played Roseanne's husband, "Dan," experienced a heart attack (very realistic given the actor John Goodman's girth) while attending the television wedding of his TV daughter. In subsequent episodes, "Dan" was supposed to be on a low-fat diet and a regular exercise program. He couldn't do it. He lied about exercising. He cheated with his food. Finally he said to Roseanne, "I can't live on this food." Well, that is a choice—one can always elect to kill oneself—but more significantly, it is also a public outcry of a different sort. Basically, he and millions of other individuals, not necessarily in TV Land, are saying, "I don't care if I die early, or have a stroke, live like a vegetable"—excuse the choice of that word, vegetables aren't usually associated with these individuals—"or have my chest sliced open and have surgery. The food is more important, and don't even think of mentioning exercise." That is their concept of "going public."

I had a client, about fifty pounds overweight, who worked with my firm for about six months. One day he called me to say that he was light-headed, sweating, and had chest pains coming home from a golf game. I urged him to immediately get to the emergency room. He was indeed having a heart attack. Three days later he had a quintuple bypass. Three months later I bumped into him at a restaurant and asked how his cardiac rehabilitation was coming along (I was assuming he was participating). He said, "I'm not going to get all riled up about this." I, in total disbelief, said, "Well sure, it's up to you." He had a heart attack, was fortunate enough to have lived, had a successful bypass operation, which included having his chest sliced open, but no, he wasn't going to get riled up about this and take care of himself. Think about that for a moment. One wonders, what would get him riled up?

So, you publicly state your intent. You will receive varied responses. Remember, I did all your research on the competition for you in the previous chapter. When you explain your inten-

The Business Plan for the Body

tions and someone says to you, "Forget that, go on a high-protein diet to lose weight," politely explain that you would prefer to be a healthier, lean person and not an individual whose body is placed in ketosis in order to lose weight. When someone tells you, "It's all in your genes, just accept your weight," explain to them that yes, genes play a role, but your genes *and* your behavior got you to your present weight. You are now going to change your behavior. When someone else tells you to forget all that exercise and just diet, explain the benefits of your program and the necessity of exercise, especially strength and resistance exercise. Do you see the value of our research? In the past you might have been enticed by the "quick fix" or by the numerous fallacies you may have heard, or even believed. Now you know better. Remember, you are the man or the woman with the plan.

TRUST YOUR RESEARCH

STRATEGIC ACTION PLAN

We reiterated our mission statement. We've reviewed the competition. We are now "going public" with our business plan. "Going public" creates a totally new environment, within which we will now function. Just as public corporations face constant pressure from their shareholders to succeed with their business plans, we, too, will now expose ourselves to pressure to succeed. The human mind is a complex entity, and the line between its conscious and subconscious boundaries many times blurs. That's why proclaiming your goals to your spouse, friends, children, coworkers, restaurant waiters, and others around you will keep any subconscious desires you might possess in check. Yes, you will be subjecting yourself to a degree of pressure, but pressure is necessary. Pressure will keep your business plan headed in the right direction. Make it a positive force.

You've tried in private, now you're entering the public arena. Sure it's scary, but you now have a plan. You have *The Business Plan for the Body,* you're taking it public and you're going to be a smashing public success.

As Queen Vicky said, "We're not interested in the possibilities of defeat." She wasn't defeated. Nor will you be.

THE MANAGEMENT TEAM

4 *Your Key Players*

When I first meet a client for my $10,000-a-week program, I ask that the spouse or significant other be present. At one memorable meeting, I met with overwhelming hostility from the client's wife. She virtually disagreed with everything I had to say. She was overweight and quite threatened by the fact that her husband was doing my program and was very serious about losing weight and improving his health. She had absolutely no interest in my eating and exercise advice for herself. When I had time alone with my client the following day, I asked him, "What are you going to do about your wife's objection to this plan?" He said, "I do a lot of things my wife objects to. This will just be another." That's a shame. If just the fact that he was trying to get on plan stirred up issues between them, just think what is going to happen when he succeeds at the plan.

On the other hand, I have a thirty-year-old woman who has been a smashing success. She is five feet three inches tall and started my program at 130 pounds. Five months later she is down to 115.5 pounds. She faxes me her food diaries and is consistent with her workouts. But the biggest reason for her success is her husband. Granted, in the beginning he was skeptical, but once she got rolling, he became an enormous help. He compliments her all the time, tells her how great she looks,

"You're only as good as the people you hire."

RAY KROC,
FOUNDER OF
MCDONALD'S

encourages her to exercise, surprised her with more exercise equipment on her birthday, takes the bread basket politely off the table, and basically gives her so much support. I frequently ask her if he would like a job. He is exactly the type of person I would want on my team, and a big reason why she is such a success.

You have decided to get into the weight-loss business. You have researched the competition and determined who is getting it right and who is getting it wrong. You went public with your intent. Now the time has come to assemble and educate your next component—"The Management Team."

The management team is essential to the success of your business plan. Most companies have a small group of senior executives who both create and implement the course of the business plan. Numerous publicly traded stocks are bought and sold both on the basis of earnings and on the perception of who comprises the corporate management team. A *Wall Street Journal* article in December 1999 discussed the General Electric Corporation's concern regarding the departure of its current CEO, Jack F. Welch, Jr. The article noted that Mr. Welch will be retiring in approximately sixteen months. Yes, that's right, his retirement was still sixteen months in the future but the company was already trying to prepare Wall Street for this change in the management team. That's how important Mr. Welch was perceived to be to the success of General Electric. Remember how Apple Computer stock rose when Steven Jobs initially returned to head the company? What do you think would happen to the stock if Steven Jobs once again retired?

In the preceding chapter I urged you to *go public*. I also explained that when a company is preparing an initial public offering (IPO), one of the most valuable opportunities a potential investor or analyst has is to attend a road show, a breakfast, lunch, or dinner meeting where the management team is presented to potential investors. Investors and analysts would agree, the strength of the management team is frequently a significant factor in their decision to invest.

ASSEMBLE AND EDUCATE YOUR MANAGEMENT TEAM

What do these examples have in common? All illustrate how critical the management team is to the success of the venture. The same applies to you. When I do my intensive $10,000-a-week program, I know that the time spent with the client's management team is one of the most valuable services I provide. I sit down, usually for at least an hour, with each person the client comes in contact with on a daily basis, and fully explain the development and implementation of the plan. Since you do not have me to complete this task, you have to learn how to do it on your own. The following is a road map for doing just that.

First, identify the current members of your senior management team. Start with the key player, or the person closest to you. This may be your spouse, partner, parent, sibling, or best friend. Sit him or her down and be calm. Do not do this over the phone or in a rush. It must be done in person and conveyed slowly. State your mission statement. Be clear, once again tell him or her you are embarking on a new business venture. Since you already went public, this person will be aware of your intention. Be specific as you explain the plan and the role you are asking him or her to play. Give details.

IDENTIFY YOUR KEY PLAYERS

Just saying "I am going to try to lose weight" is not enough. Explain why. Make it clear to the person that he or she is the most important person in your life and subsequently will be key to the success of your plan. You are going to make many changes in your life, and you want each member of your management team to understand your needs and goals. This will be an ongoing process, so explain that there will be many adjustments as you proceed.

Next, meet with the person with whom you spend the greatest amount of your time. This might not be the person with whom you live. However, this individual clearly will be a member of your senior management team. This may be an executive assistant, a business associate, a best friend, a coworker, a family member, or an individual who helps you in your home or with your children. Same rules apply. Sit this person down and explain the components of the plan. Tell them that you need their help and support. Let them in on the fact that you already had this conversation with the key player on your team. This will let them know how serious you are about your mission.

If applicable, the next environment to include would be your office. Clearly, your closest coworker or your administrative assistant should be included on the senior management team. You may decide to include your boss, who I bet will be thrilled

The Business Plan for the Body

you are going "on plan." Don't forget, one of the residual benefits of going on plan is increased productivity and creativity. I don't know of a single employer who wouldn't want an employee to look better, feel better, perform better, and possess more energy. Study after study has demonstrated that healthy people take fewer sick days and file fewer health care claims.

Once you have assembled the senior management team, proceed to include the ancillary players. Your goal is to continue to widen your management team. The whole "corporation" is going to be on board with your plan. In your home, additional family members who live with you, and any support staff such as a housekeeper, should be included. Don't forget to include the kids. I receive my best "inside" information on aberrant client behavior from their children. Most run up to me at the door and say, "Mommy ate cake for breakfast." Kids love to police. Empower them. Including the kids in your management team not only provides them with information on healthy eating habits and exercise, but sets a good example as well.

DON'T FORGET TO INCLUDE THE KIDS

For some of you, your management team may be composed of a handful of people, such as a spouse, parent, a few coworkers, and a few friends. For others this may take some time, as you have many people involved in your life. But regardless of the size, make sure your team will help you remain confident, strong, committed, and powerful. Remember, *you are the man with the plan.*

Who is your "Director of Purchasing" or the person who does the majority of the grocery shopping in your home? Sit down with this person, or by yourself, if it's you, and develop an eating plan for the coming week (more on this in Chapter 6). You determine what meals and snacks you will eat at home and what you will eat when you go out. Next, decide what to buy for the home and where you are going to go when you eat out. Nothing is left to chance. You will be organized, and therefore increase your ability to have a successful eating week. In other words, you will be in control of your calories in, plus you're managing "the numbers," which we will explore in subsequent chapters.

You should develop a standard weekly grocery list with your Director of Purchasing. Keep it in either a daily planner, computer, or personal digital assistant (PDA). Each week, go to the store (or use the Internet, phone, or fax) and make your purchases by following the list. Your "supplies" will be taken care of without you having to think about it. This is a great way to set a weekly plan in motion, and you only have to modify it infrequently. This definitely takes the air out of all the people who say "eating healthy takes so much time and energy."

Certain aspects of your meetings will be simple. Let's say you have lots of snacks, chips, cookies, and candy at home. Simply say, "We have to make some adjustments in our snacks. We have to include fresh fruit, cut-up vegetables, and other healthy alternatives." When it comes to meals, make sure the words "steamed," "poached," or "baked" replace the words "fried," "sauteed," and "breaded." Again, in your presentation, be prepared to compromise on certain delicate issues. If you regularly order Chinese food with family or friends, simply ask for an additional order of steamed vegetables with chicken or shrimp. That's not so hard.

BE WILLING TO COMPROMISE

The following is a suggested format for each of your meetings:

MEETING FORMAT

1. **Clearly articulate your mission statement.** In addition to the statement, give examples of what brought you to this decision. Be specific.

2. **Summarize** *The Business Plan for the Body.* Use the business plan analogy to illustrate how you are modeling your program on a comprehensive business plan. Read the book chapter titles out loud. Those who have ever read or written a business plan will possess a clear understanding of the structure, but others will also easily comprehend your strategy.

3. **Articulate your goals.** Many of these may be personalized (as I urged you to do in your mission statement), such as "I want to be a size x by y." Others may be weight goals, such as "I want to weigh x by y." Others may be event goals, such as "I want to participate in a race on a set date." Whatever it may be, set

quantifiable goals and be open about them. Remember, public pressure is a powerful motivating force.

4. **Be very clear that you need their help.** Most people will not deny you help. If the people you are speaking with are also out of shape, you might encourage them to participate in some aspect of the plan. Or let them know that if they want to go "on plan," you will be there for them. Generally, the only time someone will deny you help is when it involves money. Apart from money, you should be fine.

5. **Be very clear about the role you are asking them to play.** If the individual you are talking to is your Friday night pizza buddy, then tell him or her that you still want to spend Friday evenings together, but the venue will have to change. If this person frequently makes your favorite pie, then explain that you love the pie but want to save it for a few special occasions. Don't lie, don't soft-pedal, don't apologize. This is your life. This is your plan. You are going to succeed.

6. **Ask your team not to judge.** I know, almost every one of you has tried to lose weight in the past. Many of your team may have experienced your past ups and downs. Again, if you make clear to your management team that this is not a fad diet, not an impulse purchase, not a gimmick but a real program, you will get a far more favorable response. Be serious, and they will respond in kind.

7. **Describe the comprehensive nature of the plan.** Explain that you are going to approach your program by addressing all three variables: eating, exercise, and the right mind-set.

At this point, I know what you are thinking. You are saying to yourself "Right, like my husband, wife, or partner will be on my team. Their behavior is worse than mine. How are they going to help me?" Well, this will depend on your delivery. Don't be defensive. Don't be judgmental. Don't cop an attitude. Instead, clearly lay out your needs and how you hope they will be key players and part of your team. The more important you make them feel to the success of your plan, the more they will be apt to comply and provide assistance.

Think about that issue for a moment. Look someone in the eye and say, "I need your help, you are important to my success." Do you really think they will say no? Try it. I bet you will be surprised by their response. Again, so much of their response will be dependent upon your delivery. Be sincere. Be vulnerable. Most people will respond to a cry for help. And remember, most of these people are individuals who already care about you.

Keep in mind, these conversations must take place in person. Don't even think about the phone, e-mail, or any other form of nonpersonal communication. Presence has power. Use it. Convince your team that this time is different. This time you will succeed with your plan.

We had a client participating in a program we provide that we call the "Ten, Ten, Ten." This is different from the intensive $10,000 one-week program, though, as you can see, I do have a strong attachment to that ten grand number. In this ten-week program, we fitness-train clients for ten hours a week for ten weeks, guarantee that they lose a minimum of ten pounds, and charge them $10,000. At the end of the ten weeks, if they haven't shed a minimum of ten pounds, we will refund their money—if they pass a lie detector test stating they never varied from the plan. To date we have never had to administer the test and everyone has lost over ten pounds, some as much as thirty pounds. They stayed on their plan. To illustrate, one of our clients who participated in this program, a woman in her early thirties, likes to eat out with her husband. We called the restaurants she selected and reviewed their menus. I helped her order and stay on plan. We had to eliminate a few places because they just had nothing appropriate on the menu, but for the most part the husband and wife compromised on restaurant choices and she was able to appease her spouse and stay on plan. These days, most restaurants will prepare foods according to your specifications. Don't be shy or intimidated. Ask. By the way, she lost twenty-four pounds in the ten weeks. She looks great. And wouldn't you know, her husband also lost weight, without even trying, and is thrilled.

Here is another idea. Bring the whole team together. You might host a breakfast, lunch, or dinner and get as many of your team together as possible. This might give everyone a chance to hear your plan and better determine what role each person will play. Make it fun. Create esprit de corps. Give everyone a title, such as, Director of Caloric Intake; Vice President, Fitness; Chief Financial Officer (the person who weighs you); Communications Manager (the person who calls your lunch buddy and relays the information on what you ate to your dinner pal); or whatever titles you want to create. Give your team a common sense of purpose. You are going to lose weight, and they are going to help you make it happen. Make everyone realize you are all in this business together. This is a united, corporate-wide endeavor. Believe me, your management team is a huge key to your success with the plan. They will support you physically, as they help you actually design and execute the plan, and emotionally, as they give you ongoing encouragement and focus.

HOST A TEAM MEETING

COPING WITH NEGATIVISM

One word of caution when assembling a management team. You may have to make some deletions—that is, omit or "fire" someone. This is not easy. If someone is unable to be a member of your team, get some distance. It may only be for a brief period of time, but it might be imperative to your success. You need strength to stay on plan, and negative people require a lot of your energy. Some people may be negative, dismissive, and uncooperative from the start. Give them a chance, but establish your limits. Many people are threatened by change. In Chapter 10, "I Did It, I Did It," I explore many of the responses you may receive when you are a success in the weight-loss business. Many of those responses are similar to the ones you now may be receiving as you announce your intent to go into the weight-loss business. A spouse may think, "He (or she) will leave me if they lose weight," or a friend might think if you lose weight, you will no longer have eating in common. Only you can decide how to handle these situations. Just be prepared.

If someone says, "You'll never lose weight. Who are you kidding?" then look them in the eye and say, "This time is different because I have a plan, *The Business Plan for the Body.*" Prove them wrong, lose the weight. I love the saying "The best revenge is living well." It applies to your new plan and subsequent success. Losing weight will prove to them that you are serious with your intent.

Now don't get me wrong, I am not telling you to divorce a noncompliant spouse, but you will have an uphill battle and need to be prepared for their lack of cooperation.

STRATEGIC ACTION PLAN

Assemble and educate your management team. Similar to a business organization, the better the team, the higher the probability of success and profitability derived from the plan. You are going to prepare for and schedule meetings with the key people in your home, office, and other relevant environments. You've gone public, so they know your intentions and now will know the specifics and what role you will ask each of them to play. Phase one of your plan is almost complete. What is left is to delve into the numbers. Then we take action.

You are on your way. You are in charge. You are the leader.

The Business Plan for the Body

THE FINANCIALS

5 *Understand the Numbers*

There is a woman with whom I occasionally chat in the elevator of my office building who is always on some kind of crazy eating program. Here is her latest. She is convinced that if she does not eat anything after 6:00 P.M., she will lose weight. I try to explain to her that if she overeats during the day and takes in too many calories, it does not matter what time she stops eating, she has eaten too much. The body does not say, "Oh, since you stopped eating by 5:00 P.M., I will reward you with weight loss." Doesn't happen. A calorie is a calorie—NO MATTER WHERE OR WHEN IT IS CONSUMED. Next you'll be reading and listening to testimonials telling you that some rooms in your home are more conducive to weight loss than others. I can hear it now, "If I eat in the den, I don't gain as much as I do when I eat in the living room!"

There is a man I know who claims that if he eats anything over 800 calories, he gains weight. Every time he tells me this, I smile and nod. I have witnessed this gentleman at dinner parties and benefits. He eats everything in sight. How could he possibly believe that he is eating only 800 calories? Obviously, he is not doing the necessary math. I would say the number he is consuming per day is closer to 3,800 calories.

> "As a rule, he or she who has the most information will have the greatest success in life."
>
> **DISRAELI**

At this point, the research and development phase of your program requires one final step, examining the "financials." To succeed in the weight-loss business, it is imperative to review specific financial components, commonly known as the "numbers." Just as corporations estimate revenues and expenses to project earnings, you will begin inputting the appropriate numbers into the following equation:

The Weight-Loss Equation
Calories in minus calories out = Your body weight

The first part of this equation, the calories in, is simply the number of calories you consume on a daily basis. The second part of the equation, the calories out, comes from your metabolism and daily caloric burning. Metabolism is truly the single most misunderstood function of the body. What is this process called metabolism? Simply put, metabolism is the process of energy expenditure. You have to look at your present body weight as a function of energy in (calories) minus energy out (calories). Calories are units of energy that our body burns in many ways. Right now, as you sit reading this book, you are burning calories. How can that be? This occurs because your body is operating at all times. It never stops. You are breathing, your cells are rejuvenating, your food is digesting, your brain is functioning. All of these internal activities and others require energy, or calories. Let's get this definition straight once again. A calorie is a unit of energy. Our body uses energy to perform each and every function. But when a unit of energy is consumed and not spent, it is stored. The name for that stored unit of energy is called *body fat*.

DO THE NUMBERS

Your body is in motion even when you are sleeping. I bet you thought you had to be on a treadmill to burn calories? Wrong! Think about an idling car. The car is turned on, the motor is running, but it isn't going anywhere. Is the car burning gas? Absolutely, in the same way the body is burning calories, even at rest. You can turn a car off, but the body's metabolism doesn't turn off until you do; in other words, until you die.

CALORIES ARE UNITS OF ENERGY

Metabolism is composed of three major components and numerous minor ones. Let's examine what constitutes your body's major metabolic components.

The Business Plan for the Body

BASAL METABOLIC RATE

We all have a basal metabolic rate, which I will refer to as BMR. The BMR is basically the number of calories our body would need each day if we never—I repeat, never—got out of bed, stayed awake for approximately sixteen hours, and slept for approximately eight. Even though you are lying down, your body requires a certain amount of energy to perform essential physiological functions such as breathing, neurological functioning, heartbeat, digestion, and cell formation, in addition to many others. Sixty to 70 percent of the calories you use on a daily basis are devoted to those functions.

METABOLISM IS THE PROCESS OF ENERGY EXPENDITURE

How do we determine BMR? In the early twentieth century, studies of basal metabolic rate were conducted at the Nutrition Laboratory of the Carnegie Institution of Washington. The research was led by Francis G. Benedict. The name of this widely accepted equation to determine basal metabolic rate is the Harris-Benedict equation. Note that I have changed this equation from metric to U.S. measurements. Now get out your calculator (I hope you realize every successful businessperson owns one). I want you to input your weight, height, and age into the following equations:

Women
$$661 + (4.38 \times \text{weight in pounds}) + (4.38 \times \text{height in inches}) - (4.7 \times \text{age}) = \text{BMR}$$
Men
$$67 + (6.24 \times \text{weight in pounds}) + (12.7 \times \text{height in inches}) - (6.9 \times \text{age}) = \text{BMR}$$

Let me use myself as an example. I am forty years old, six feet tall—or seventy-two inches—and weigh 175 pounds:

$$\text{Jim Karas: } 67 + (6.24 \times 175) + (12.7 \times 72) - (6.9 \times 40) = \text{BMR}$$
$$\text{or}$$
$$67 + 1{,}092 + 914.4 - 276 = 1{,}797.40$$

So, on a daily basis, I burn 1,797.4 calories if I stay in bed all day. If you are having difficulty with this equation, please go to my website at *www.businessplanforthebody.com* and simply plug in your weight, height, and age. Let's now examine the impact of activity on one's metabolism.

ACTIVITY

Activity is the second component of metabolism. It can account for 20 to 30 percent of your metabolism. To determine your additional calories burned through activity, it is necessary to use a multiplier. To determine the total amount of calories from *basal metabolism* and *activity* you require each day to stay at your present weight, multiply the following numbers by your BMR:

ACTIVITY MULTIPLIER

Sedentary	1.15 multiplier
Light Activity (normal, everyday activities)	1.3 multiplier
Moderately Active (exercise 3 to 4 times a week)	1.4 multiplier
Very Active (exercise more than 4 times a week)	1.6 multiplier
Extremely Active (exercise 6 to 7 times a week)	1.8 multiplier

Personally, I consider myself a very active person, as I exercise five hours a week, so I take my 1,797.4 resting metabolic number and multiply it by the very active multiplier, or 1.6:

$$1,797.4 \text{ (BMR)} \times 1.6 \text{ (very active)}$$
$$= 2,875.84 \text{ Total Calories Burned Each Day}$$

So, on a daily basis, my weight will not change if I eat approximately 2,875.84 calories each day.

I know this is tedious, but it is necessary to the "financials" of our plan. For those of you who didn't read or skimmed the introduction to this book, I am a graduate of the University of Pennsylvania's Wharton School of Business with an economics degree. I have been successful in the weight-loss business for thirteen years because I approach weight loss by the numbers. You *must* complete this equation. It will be an eye-opening experience to see the data. Remember, numbers don't lie, they are reality. Would you invest in a company that stated, "We don't look at numbers. Just take our word for it." I would hope not. Why do you think income statements, balance sheets,

The Business Plan for the Body

and the like exist? Use the information and profit from the data.

For just a moment take a look at the multipliers for each activity level. If you go from a light, active multiplier (normal, everyday activities) of 1.3 and become a moderately active multiplier (exercise three to four times a week), your daily caloric burning will go up by 7.7 percent. If you go from a light, active multiplier (normal, everyday activities) of 1.3 to a very active multiplier (exercise more than four times a week), your daily caloric burning will go up 23 percent. Finally, and you know where I am headed, if you go from a light, active multiplier (normal, everyday activities) of 1.3 to an extremely active (exercise six to seven times a week), your daily caloric burning will go up by a whopping 38.5 percent. These are huge increases in the body's ability to burn calories. Once again, this point should illustrate how exercise is essential to maximizing the number of "calories out" in our equation. Exercise is essential to weight loss by the numbers.

Now, take a look at both equations. Notice how much smaller the numbers are for women than for men. Women have to accept the fact that they can't eat the same number of calories as most men and lose weight. I strongly believe that menus should include a men's portion and a women's portion. Whatever happened to the "petite" filet from the 1960s? If women eat as much as most men, they are not going to be successful in the weight-loss business. I started my fitness training business in 1988 with a half-dozen women, five feet three inches tall and under, who were struggling with their weight. They were frustrated, but through my program learned that they must be aware of their calorie intake and consistently exercise. If you are a woman, don't be discouraged. You can lose weight and feel great. It simply takes a little more fine-tuning than it does for men.

INCREASE YOUR MULTIPLIER

Observe the following. One man, one woman, both forty-five years of age, five feet eight inches tall, 150 pounds. Input these numbers into the respective BMR equations and see the results on page 64. Therefore, a man's basal metabolic rate is approximately 150 calories a day higher. This difference is the function of these variables:

Women 661 + (4.38 × weight in pounds) + (4.38 × height in inches)
– (4.7 × age) = BMR

Men 67 + (6.24 × weight in pounds) + (12.7 × height in inches) – (6.9
× age) = BMR

Man: 1,556.10 calories a day   Woman: 1,404.34 calories a day

- *Genetically, men have more muscle than women; subsequently their metabolisms are higher.*
- *Men have 3 percent essential body fat (the minimum their bodies need to function properly) and women have 12 percent essential body fat, primarily because of their reproductive organs and breasts.*

Therefore, a man's basal metabolic rate will be higher than a woman's, though I should point out that a woman's basal metabolic rate is higher during menstruation.

One more important point regarding the equation. Realize that the higher your body weight, the higher your basal metabolic rate. This is a point I constantly make to overweight individuals. If you are overweight, you have a higher basal metabolic rate and require more calories on a daily basis to maintain your overweight status than a thinner individual. Simply by overeating, which every overweight person does, you actually are increasing your metabolism. The skinnies of the world are the ones who should use the "bad" metabolism excuse, but they don't need to. Let me repeat, if you are overweight you have to consistently keep overeating in order to keep the weight on. If you stopped overeating, you would lose weight. Simple arithmetic. The equation doesn't lie.

Allow me to elaborate on this point. Say you have two people, same sex, height, age, and exercise habits, but one weighs twenty pounds more than the other. Clearly, the heavier individual requires more calories each day than the lighter one to maintain the higher weight. Look at the components of the equation. The higher your weight, the more calories you need on a daily basis to maintain that weight. But if the heavier individual reduces his or her caloric intake and eats the same amount

MOST MEN
BURN MORE
CALORIES THAN
WOMEN

The Business Plan for the Body

of calories as a lighter one, over time the heavier individual will lose weight and weigh the same as the lighter individual.

There is yet a third component to metabolism, and that involves the food you eat and the digestion of that food. What you eat *and* when you eat can have a significant impact on your body's metabolism.

DIGESTION

Digestion accounts for 7 to 13 percent of your metabolism. Think about that. You can alter your metabolism by what, when, and how much you are eating.

HOW MUCH ARE YOU EATING?

If you are overweight, you are overeating. Your digestive system is working around the clock to process all the food. When you overeat (think Thanksgiving dinner, which should happen once a year but in many households happens once a day) your body speeds up in order to blow off the additional calories. That is why you are so exhausted after the meal. All of your body's energy is going to digest the dinner. Reflect on that. Overeating actually speeds up your metabolism, because your body is working to keep you at "fighting" weight. In other words, your body does not want to be overweight.

This is the point I made earlier with regard to overweight individuals who claim they have "bad," meaning slow, metabolisms. In fact, they are overeating and that increases their metabolism because they are forcing their bodies to work harder to digest all the additional food. Unfortunately, overweight people are eating so much more than they require on a daily basis that even with that metabolic boost they are experiencing, they continue to gain weight. *Their behavior is overriding the body's natural defense mechanism.*

DIGESTION BOOSTS METABOLISM

WHAT ARE YOU EATING?

It's now appropriate to explore *what* you are eating. There are three food categories: *carbohydrate, protein,* and *fat.* According to the American Medical Association:

Carbohydrate includes all starches and sugars. They are the body's main source of energy. Each gram of carbohydrate provides 4 calories. Most foods contain carbohydrates. Sugar is a carbohydrate. The main sugar in food is sucrose, which is white and brown sugar, while the other sugars are lactose (found in milk) and fructose (found in fruits and vegetables). Starches are a more complex form of carbohydrate and includes beans, breads, cereals, pasta, and potatoes.

Protein is the body's building material for muscle, skin, bone, and hair. Protein is made up of a chain of amino acids. Each gram of protein provides 4 calories. The body uses proteins to make antibodies, or disease-fighting chemicals, and certain hormones such as insulin, which serve as chemical messengers in the body. Proteins include meat, fish, poultry, dairy products, eggs, legumes, and nuts.

Fat is divided into three categories. Saturates, often called "bad" fat, monounsaturated fat, and polyunsaturated fat. Each gram of fat provides 9 calories, which is over twice that contained in a gram of carbohydrate or protein. Fat does pack a lot of energy, but if not expended, will become body fat.

How do these three categories affect metabolism? Protein generally is the most complex food and subsequently the most difficult to digest. It stays in the stomach longer than carbohydrates and most fats; therefore, you will have a physical feeling of fullness for a longer period of time when you consume protein. As you will see in the eating plan described in Chapter 6, a little bit of protein should be included with every meal. Now don't start with the high-protein diets again. We eliminated that approach to weight loss in Chapter 2. If you have to, go back and reread that section. Fruits and vegetables, on the other hand, pass very quickly through the stomach and the colon as they are high in fiber. And remember, the majority of vitamins and minerals in food comes from fruits and vegetables. That is why I constantly advocate eating so many of them.

Remember, too, fruits and vegetables are carbohydrates. All the talk about eliminating "carbs" from one's diet mostly pertains to bread, pasta, and rice, or other densely caloric carbohydrates. That does not include fruits and vegetables. They should never be avoided.

I am frequently asked, "Are calories from fat harder to burn than calories from carbohydrates?" There really is no difference in how fat and carbohydrates are burned, but there is a difference in how they are stored. If you were to eat 100 excess carbohydrate calories, those 100 calories must first be converted to triglycerides, which are made up of a glycerol molecule and three fatty acids. This process uses about 25 percent of the excess calories consumed, so in our example, that would translate to only 75 excess calories stored as body fat. On the other hand, if you were to eat 100 excess fat calories, the process of turning fat into body fat requires only 3 percent of the excess fat calories consumed, so you would store 97 calories as body fat. Obviously, if you are going to overeat, doing the former is preferable to the latter, though I thought we agreed we were out of the overeating business and into the weight-loss business.

WHEN ARE YOU EATING?

With regards to *when* you consume your food, the amount of time between meals is a significant issue. If you eat one big meal a day, as many people I know do, then for over twenty-two hours a day your body is in starvation mode. It thinks that it has to slow down to keep you alive since you are not eating, the same phenomenon we previously discussed that occurs when you fast or go on a highly restrictive low-calorie diet. Then, once a day, you accost the body with food. Not smart. You need to space your food as best you can throughout the day, which keeps your metabolism up. But keep in mind, eating throughout the day is not the same as *overeating* throughout the day. Remember the anecdote that introduced this chapter. That individual believed that she could eat whatever she wanted throughout the day as long as she stopped eating by a certain time. Now stop a moment and think about how ridiculous this sounds. In this scenario, not only is she placing the body in starvation mode by ceasing to eat by a certain time, but accosting her body with food the rest of the time.

Our bodies are very smart. That is why OptiFast, a liquid protein diet (Oprah's very public first diet) and other similar crash diets did not work—because they caused the body to go into starvation mode. I know I explained this before but it bears repeating. If you drink or eat a very restricted diet, say 400 to 500 calories a day, your body thinks that you are being starved to death and slows your metabolism in order to keep you alive. An important point to realize is that one of the ways the body slows itself down is to attack lean muscle tissue, which is the body's most "active" tissue. Using our business analogy, lean muscle is our "capital" and must be preserved. So, severe dieting is not a viable option.

NEVER SKIP MEALS

But what happens when you overeat? Just the opposite. Your body speeds up because it doesn't want to carry around extra calories stored as fat. That's right, your body is not your enemy but your number one ally. Your body does not want to be over-weight. So, stop blaming your body and start blaming your behavior.

Please note. Most crash diets, like all the ridiculous articles you read that tout "Lose Ten Pounds in Ten Days" or "The Five-Day Quick-Fix Diet" do nothing but ruin your metabolism. The following study reflects this fact.

The *Journal of American Medicine* reported a study that examined the effects of repeated cycles of weight loss and re-gain on adolescent wrestlers. High school and college wrestlers are constantly going on crash diets prior to competition in order to make a lower weight category, which their coaches believe will give them an advantage. Ultimately, they found that there was a 14 percent lower meta-bolic rate in those adolescent wrestlers who repeatedly lost and regained weight versus those who did not. Even at a very young age, the meta-bolic rate was significantly impaired. Just think about how this affects most of us who are considerably beyond adolescence.

PRESERVE LEAN MUSCLE TISSUE AT ALL COSTS

Historically, prior to the industrial revolution, excess weight was not an issue. Excess weight is not an issue in most third world countries, where the problem is more apt to be one of starvation. Your body wants to be at a lower weight, and once you begin my program you will be amazed by the results as your body cooperates.

Okay, you are still convinced that you have a bad metabolism? You're a special case. You are unique. You are not like the other 99.999999999999999 percent of the population. Well, the following will dissuade you of that notion.

VARIABLES THAT AFFECT OUR METABOLISM

GENES

Many people blame their supposed "bad" metabolism on their genes. They make statements such as, "My mother and father are overweight so I am doomed." We established in Chapter 2 that 25 percent of your body weight is determined by your genes, the rest is determined by your environment and behavior. At present there is a great deal of medical research being conducted on the role genes play in determining our body weight, composition, and metabolism. Two people starting at the same height, weight, age, body fat content, and fitness level, if put on the same weight-loss program, will lose weight at different speeds, but they will both *lose weight*. It might be somewhat more difficult for some individuals than others, but that's life. If you want to look and feel good, you have to work at it as you do with all aspects of your life.

Think about yourself. What comes easily to you? Maybe it's sports, or math, or an ability to program your VCR. I personally have a very good memory (I can remember the phone numbers of almost every one of my clients—home, office, and cellular) but I am pathetic when I attempt to speak a foreign language. People always comment on how good my memory is and similarly shudder when I attempt to speak French or Greek.

We know from extensive medical research that the child of an alcoholic does have a greater genetic predisposition to also become an alcoholic. But that does not mean all such children will become alcoholics. They can give in to their genetic programming or do something about it. Being aware of genetic tendencies can prevent them from becoming reality. Keep in mind, the word "predisposition" is different from the word "predetermined." Predisposition, you have a choice; predetermined, basically, is a fait accompli. You are not predetermined to be overweight. You might be predis-

ONLY 25 PERCENT OF BODY WEIGHT IS DETERMINED BY GENES

posed, but you are not predetermined to be overweight. You have the choice.

Most genetic research deals with the obese and morbidly obese, not your friend Jane who is fifty-three years old, five feet five inches tall, 125 pounds in college, and now weighs 155 pounds on a "good" day. If you never had a weight problem and now do, don't even think of blaming your genes. Jane's weight gain is behavior-related and not genetic.

THYROID FUNCTION

What function does the thyroid perform? Basically, think of the thyroid as the battery of your body's metabolism. In a car, if the battery is low, many of the automobile's functions will not work at full capacity. Similarly, if your thyroid is not producing enough hormone, many of the following symptoms may arise: weight gain; difficulty losing weight; fatigue; dry, coarse hair or hair loss; abnormal menstrual cycles; depression; constipation; cold intolerance; pale skin; memory loss; or decreased sexual libido. The severity and number of symptoms will vary with the amount of thyroid dysfunction.

Eleven million Americans do suffer from the most common type of thyroid illness, termed hypothyroidism. The majority are women or the elderly. Note, this number represents an extremely small percent of the American population. Of the eleven million, approximately half are aware they have the disorder and actively seek medical assistance. I know you are convinced that you are one of this small percentage of individuals. Okay, if you think you may be one of the eleven million, go take a simple blood test, as I urged you in Chapter 2, which any physician can administer. Then stop using thyroid as an excuse. If there is an abnormality, once medicated, the thyroid can function normally. But stop for one moment and be honest about your behavior. I can't tell you how many of my clients have repeatedly gone for blood tests for thyroid dysfunction. They've stuffed themselves with cheese, oil, cake, candy, huge bowls of pasta, and similar "high caloric" goodies, but insist that their thyroid is the reason for their weight problem. Denial runs very deep in our culture.

PREDISPOSITION AND PREDETERMINED ARE NOT THE SAME

In addition, if you begin taking thyroid medication and don't have an underactive thyroid (I actually know people who have

The Business Plan for the Body

convinced their doctor they desperately need it), then you will succeed in *creating* a thyroid problem. This occurs because the thyroid will shut down since the body senses there is too much thyroid hormone in the system inasmuch as you are unnecessarily supplementing the body with medication.

LEAN MUSCLE TISSUE

Lean muscle tissue is simply muscle. Muscle is critically important to your metabolism because it is the body's most active tissue.

What is meant by active tissue? Simple. Muscle requires more feeding, or calories, than other tissue throughout the day and night to survive, therefore making it the most active tissue in our bodies. We have established that a calorie is a unit of energy, so think of muscles as requiring lots of energy to survive. Or think of muscles as "big spenders," since they expend a lot of calories staying active. So by increasing the amount of muscle on your body, you are forcing your body to be a big caloric spender. That will increase the second part, the calories out, in our equation. How can you increase your lean muscle tissue? *Only through strength and resistance training!*

Strength and resistance training is the most effective method of exercise in order to build muscle. By creating resistance through the use of free weights, weight-training machines, elastic tubing, or your own body weight, a muscle is challenged to perform an activity beyond its current strength level. Challenging a muscle stimulates a muscle to grow, producing more lean muscle tissue. An increase in lean muscle tissue is essential to your success in the weight-loss business. Most cardiovascular exercises, such as walking, running, stair climbing, and biking do very little if anything to increase your lean muscle tissue. Only in the embryonic stages of a cardiovascular program will a slight increase in lean muscle tissue occur. One would have to perform cardiovascular exercise at Olympian levels in order to contribute to an increase in the body's lean muscle tissue. So stop believing all the crazy infomercials that hawk cardiovascular equipment, such as the Healthrider, which claim to be "building lean muscle tissue" or "improving tone throughout your body." Only progressive strength and resistance training gets the job done, and remem-

> LEAN MUSCLE TISSUE IS CREATED THROUGH STRENGTH AND RESISTANCE TRAINING

ber to note this important term, *progression,* which will be extensively discussed in Chapter 9.

How great is the impact of an increase in lean muscle tissue on our numbers? Recent studies indicate that one pound of lean muscle tissue can burn between 35 and 50 calories per day. Just think about how those numbers will add up over time. And just for the record, a pound of fat only burns 2 to 3 calories a day. No, that is not a typographical error; a pound of fat only burns 2 to 3 calories per pound per day, while a pound of muscle burns 35 to 50 calories per pound per day.

Look at the significant number of calories expended by building lean muscle tissue through strength and resistance training:

- **Add one pound of lean muscle tissue through strength training, you will burn an additional 50 calories a day**

- **50 calories a day for 365 days equals 18,250 calories a year**

- **18,250 calories, divided by 3,500 calories (one pound of body weight), equals 5.2 pounds of weight loss a year**

Or consider the impact of five additional pounds of lean muscle tissue:

- **Add five pounds of lean muscle tissue through strength training, you will burn an additional 250 calories a day**

- **250 calories a day for 365 days equals 91,250 calories a year**

- **91,250 calories, divided by 3,500 calories (one pound of body weight), equals 26.07 pounds of weight loss a year**

Think about that for a moment. Five pounds of lean muscle tissue can burn over twenty-six pounds each and every year you maintain the muscle.

There are additional reasons why lean muscle tissue is so important to maintain and increase. After the age of twenty, the average person loses about seven pounds of lean muscle every ten years. That equates to a loss of seven-tenths of a pound of muscle a year. While this number may not seem significant, it is when you consider that you begin losing muscle at the age of twenty. For women, the bad news is that during and after menopause, the average woman will lose one pound of muscle per year, or ten pounds of muscle every ten years. Think about that. Without regular strength

MUSCLES ARE BIG CALORIC SPENDERS

The Business Plan for the Body

training, menopausal and postmenopausal women will require 35 to 50 fewer calories per day, per year.

Recall all the women you know who have gained a significant amount of weight in their forties and fifties. This occurs because of the loss of lean muscle tissue and the subsequent slowing of the metabolism. Women must strength-train, it is not an option. Adding lean muscle tissue is the only way to increase a woman's metabolism twenty-four hours a day.

WE LOSE MUSCLE EVERY YEAR

Have you ever heard someone claim that his or her muscle turned to fat or fat turned to muscle? This is impossible. Muscle and fat have nothing in common with the exception that they reside in the same body. Consider a former athlete. A young man who played football in college, six feet tall, 200 pounds, thirty-four-inch waist, and was very muscular. Years later, our athlete now weighs 250 pounds with a forty-two-inch waist and is pure fat. Did his muscle turn to fat? No. What happened was that after college he no longer played ball, ceased strength and resistance training, lost lean muscle tissue, which diminished his basal metabolic rate, but he continued the same eating habits. He experienced the same phenomenon as many menopausal women. With muscular atrophy, a reduction occurs in the basal metabolic rate and an individual will burn fewer calories twenty-four hours a day. Excess calories consumed, but not expended, become body fat. So we are clear. If you lose muscle, diminish your basal metabolic rate, and keep eating the same amount of calories, then those additional calories not expended will be stored as body fat.

Our goal is to burn the fat and build lean muscle tissue. The fat is not turning into muscle. It is being eliminated. They are two separate processes.

CLIMATE

A very hot or cold climate can force the body to work harder to cool itself down or warm itself up. I remember reading the cover of that checkout-counter staple, *The National Inquirer,* which proclaimed that you could lose ten pounds a year by lowering your thermostat in the winter and turning up your air-conditioning in the summer. While we all know this publication has been known to exaggerate, there actually is some merit to this concept, though neither I nor anyone else would be able to give an accurate number of the calories expended in these scenarios. You might save a few dollars on utility bills, but I don't think you will see great results in the mirror or on your scale.

The fact is, the body has to work overtime to regulate its internal temperature. So, if you are cold, the body will strive to return to normal temperature. Your metabolism will rise. If you are overheating, your body will similarly work to throw off the excess body heat (note, this always happens during exercise and accounts for a portion of the calories burned).

STIMULANTS

Old-fashioned diet pills were all major stimulants. These were the pills they pumped up Judy Garland with and that Patty Duke was popping in the 1960s movie *Valley of the Dolls*. The names of these pills all ended in *ine*, like dexadrine. By stimulating the body, the basal metabolism increased, not to mention the added calories you burned off as you ran around like a wild person on these drugs. Remember Fen-Phen, better known as a combination of Pondimin (fenfluramine) or Redux (dexfenfluramine) with phentermine, an amphetamine-like drug? Look at all those drugs ending in *ine*. Fen-Phen caused pulmonary hypertension and heart valve damage in numerous users and was subsequently pulled from the market.

JUST SAY NO TO DRUGS

Caffeine is also a stimulant, and some studies are showing that massive amounts of caffeine throughout the day can help in weight loss, though this is by no means recommended. Nicotine (notice another *ine*) is a major stimulant. My wife is an actress and we spend a certain amount of time around actors. Many of the tiny actresses and models smoke like chimneys. Don't forget that two of our most revered, stylish, trend-setting, sophisticated, thin icons in the twentieth century, Jacqueline Kennedy Onassis and Audrey Hepburn, smoked packs of cigarettes every day of their lives. No wonder they stayed so slim. Sadly, they both died of cancer, Jackie from non-Hodgkins lymphoma and Audrey from colon cancer.

Smoking and obesity are the number one and number two causes of death per year in the United States. Both of these are

The Business Plan for the Body

behavior-related. Both represent controllable behavior. You can elect to smoke and you can choose to allow your body to become obese. The decision is yours.

Health magazine recently reported that approximately one-third of high school students now smoke, which represents a 32 percent increase from 1991. A great many of these students do so to remain thin. Now don't go out and buy cigarettes. I'll remind you again that smoking is the number one killer in our country, with obesity right behind. Since 1964, all cigarette packages are required by law to carry the Surgeon General's warning that smoking is harmful to your health. Yet, if you can believe it, approximately 25 percent of all Americans and 33 percent of all Europeans smoke, but come on, we all know that smoking is not the answer. What you eat and whether you smoke are two controllable choices. It is within your power. I made a choice. I personally smoked for eight years of my life, loved it, but would prefer to live a longer, healthier life, and not have gross breath, yellow teeth, wrinkled skin, cancer and emphysema, smell like hell, and probably die sooner than I should. So, no smoking please. Smoking is not a cure for being overweight. It only adds to one's health problems.

SMOKING IS NOT THE ANSWER

Just a side note for those of you who are smoking and wish to stop. The biggest reason you gain weight when you quit is because your body's metabolism is changing and slowing down. Once you eliminate the stimulant, the nicotine, you will burn fewer calories on a daily basis. You also know that you do end up putting more food into your mouth when you quit smoking in order to satisfy your oral fixation. But, by quitting smoking and beginning a strength and resistance-training program, you can keep your metabolic rate elevated. Same metabolic benefit that smoking provided, but now you can forget the lung cancer, emphysema, increased risk of heart disease, bad breath, and burnt clothes. It is very doable. I know, I did it. It might take up to a year to remetabolize, and yes, an addiction is difficult to break, but not impossible. Millions have accomplished it, and so can you.

We have a terrific client in Chicago who started working with my firm at 200 pounds and who smoked. Together we decided to increase her metabolism through strength and resistance training, then to implement a weight-loss eating plan and finally to quit smoking. She did it. Two years and sixty pounds later, she is a nonsmoking, fit, energetic fifty-five-year-old, 140-pound woman. She knows she still has more weight to lose, but states the program has "changed her life." She feels stronger, healthier, and, most of all, claims she is "full of energy."

One final comment regarding the connection between smoking and weight gain. *Health* magazine recently reported the largest study ever to show a link between physical activity and giving up smoking. The study was composed of 281 sedentary female smokers between the ages of eighteen and sixty-five. The group was divided in two—one group spent two to three hours attending lectures and films, and the other spent that amount of time in the gym. The result? Twelve weeks later the active women were twice as likely to have quit smoking and had only gained half as much weight as the nonexercisers. As the researchers followed the group over the course of the next year, they noted that those who continued exercising were more likely to stay smoke-free and had avoided significant weight gain.

SMOKING/ OBESITY ARE THE NUMBER 1 & 2 CAUSES OF DEATH

FIDGETING

Can you fidget your way to weight loss? Yes. Picture all the people you know who fidget. They jiggle their legs, they tap their toes, they drum their fingers and even chew gum. These activities burn calories, and in some individuals may be the reason why they can eat more yet keep their weight down. Basically, all this fidgeting boosts their basal metabolic rate. I believe there is merit to this "fidget" factor, and a recent case study supports this belief. Researchers at the Mayo Clinic found that small scraps of movement—fidgeting, changing posture, tapping a pencil, all helped to keep weight in check. The study consisted of a group of volunteers who were fed an additional 1,000 calories per day for eight weeks. These participants were not allowed to exercise. The researchers discovered that even with the additional 1,000 calories a day, those individuals who fidgeted the most did not experience appreciable weight gain.

Here's a further illustration of the fidget factor. I live in Chicago, the home of numerous financial exchanges. I actually spent one year on the Chicago Board Options Exchange working for Merrill Lynch. I have consulted with many people who used to trade on the floor, where people stood for six to seven hours a day waving their hands, screaming and fidgeting. Once they permanently go off the floor and begin trading from their computers, they gain weight. They gain a lot of weight. Many of them call me and say, "What happened?" That's easy. Previously, on the trading floor, they burned hundreds of calories each day. Once you eliminate that activity, if you keep eating the same number of calories, you will gain weight. No way around it.

FIDGETERS BURN MORE CALORIES

How about chewing gum? Yes, recent studies have shown that gum chewing can contribute to the burning of calories, sometimes as much as 11 calories an hour. So, if you chew for, say, eight hours a day, you could burn 88 additional calories. Or you could just skip one 88-calorie cookie. Once again, the choice is yours.

Bottom line, a little fidgeting in private may be okay, but excessive fidgeting may appear to others as if you are having some sort of spasm. So be careful.

GREEN TEA

A recent study compared the effects of green tea, caffeine, and a placebo on the subject's basal metabolic rate. Each subject drank either green tea containing 375 milligrams catechins and 150 milligrams of caffeine, another beverage with 150 milligrams of caffeine, or a placebo. The results demonstrated that healthy individuals who drank green tea with every meal burned an additional 50 calories a day more than the caffeine drinkers, and 70 calories a day more than the placebo group. What caused the increase? The researchers believed the differences were caused by substances called catechins, which are antioxidants, or some other flavonoids found in green tea. However, the researchers really don't know. Bottom line, drinking two cups of green tea could help you to burn a few additional calories each day. Seventy calories a day for 365 days a year is the equivalent to 7.3 pounds of weight loss. As an added plus, drinking green tea has other potential benefits, such as reducing your risk of cancer and heart disease.

SPICY FOOD

A new study by Janet Walberg Rankin, an expert on metabolism and a professor of nutrition at Virginia Tech University, showed that eating chili peppers can elevate basal metabolism. Rankin believes that capsaicin, a compound found in jalapeño and cayenne peppers, can increase the body's release of stress hormones, like adrenaline, which increase metabolism. I'm sure we will hear more about this in the future. If you like spicy food, why not add a little of these peppers to each meal?

STRATEGIC ACTION PLAN

Do you believe in the power of the "financials"? Did you fill in the numbers to the metabolic equation and understand the significance? Do you really have a slow metabolism, "bad" genes, a thyroid problem, or is the problem your behavior? Recall our discussion regarding the difference between "predisposition" and "predetermined." Are stimulants the answer to weight loss? Heavy drugs are not, but a little green tea or caffeinated beverages might not hurt. (However, don't run out and down a half-dozen creamy cappuccinos and expect to lose weight.)

I want you to stop, think, and assess. You must be honest with yourself. You are reviewing the financial data in the privacy of your home. No one is watching. It is imperative to be honest with yourself, get out your calculator and do the math. If you refuse to work these numbers, then you are not serious about your new business venture.

Denial doesn't work. It doesn't work for anyone, and that includes you. Denial is a meaningless psychological strategy. Denial will lead to one outcome with this plan, and that's "bankruptcy."

This book is about eliminating confusion and providing you with a path. I want you to get beyond the confusion and go forth with this plan. I guarantee you will lose weight. You now have the necessary "financials" to succeed. Numbers don't lie. Your accountant would agree with me.

It's time to take action. On to Chapter 6.

Taking Action

PART II

REVENUE ALLOCATION

6
You and Your Food Diary

Recently, I was attending a dinner party at one of Chicago's toniest country clubs. I stood with a group of five other people during the cocktail hour. Three, including myself, were thin, and three were not. Frequently, when individuals find out what I do for a living, they instantly become nervous, sometimes even hostile. They also often feel compelled to discuss their weight-loss techniques. So I listened to the larger three individuals telling me about their diet and exercise programs, as they virtually inhaled thousands of calories in hors d'oeuvres, and this was before the five-course dinner. I said to the eaters, "Let me ask you, with this eating and exercise program that you are on, approximately how much weight have the three of you lost?" The group quickly disbanded. Do you think they have any idea how many calories they are taking in on a daily basis?

In the business world, when projecting the financial success of a business venture, the management team examines the components of the following basic financial equation:

"I had a wonderful evening, unfortunately this wasn't it."

GROUCHO MARX

Revenue − Expenses = Profit or Loss

Both parts of this classic equation must be explored. Apart from the craziness surrounding biotech or Internet-related stocks, traditional valuation demands that both revenues and expenses be identified to make intelligent financial projections. Similarly, as we learned from the previous chapter, "The Financials," your current weight is a function of the equation:

Calories In − Calories Out = Your Body Weight

In this chapter we are going to begin inputting the first factor of our equation, the calories in, better known to you as "food."

As you've noted, this chapter is entitled "Revenue Allocation." In our plan, your "revenue" is food, and what, when, and how much food you eat is your "allocation." You are probably saying, "Revenue allocation? I only allocate expenses." In a classic business context, that is true. A business's goal is to generate profit. Your goal is the opposite. Your goal is to generate weight loss (which is your profit). You have to allocate revenues because you want your calories in (revenues) to be low and your calories out (expenses) to be high to produce that weight loss:

CLASSIC BUSINESS EQUATION
Revenues − Expenses = Profit or Loss

The Business Plan for the Body Equation
Calories In − Calories Out = Your Body Weight

Therefore, you want to allocate your calories to keep your revenues low and exercise to keep your calories out, or expenses, high.

WHAT IS AN ALLOCATION?

Most of you already employ some aspects of allocation to your daily life, such as:

How you elect to spend your time each day. Some people work eight hours, sleep eight hours, commute to work for one hour, watch television, eat for one hour (probably more), which leaves the remaining hours for everything else. These are all allocations. As we will discuss in the next chapter, you will be committing to an additional time allocation: exercise.

How you elect to spend your money. Some people spend more on eating out, others on movies, electronic equipment, sports, clothes, or a new car. Others just spend money constantly, which I definitely equate to overeating. As a nation, Americans overeat, without considering the consequences, and just carry the excess food as body fat; similarly, they overspend, and just carry huge credit card balances. This is a major problem, and both are an example of an allocation out of whack. A weekly, monthly, or yearly spending budget is an allocation plan. You actually sit down, either alone or with your partner or spouse, and determine a comprehensive plan for spending and saving money. In my opinion, intelligent individuals budget, even if they are wealthy.

LEARN TO ALLOCATE TO LOSE WEIGHT

I am asking you to consider your eating plan as you would a monetary and time allocation. You will learn how to satisfy your body's needs, both physically and emotionally, and lose weight. We established early in this book that you know how to successfully establish an allocation to *gain* weight. Now you are going to develop and implement an eating allocation to *lose* weight.

Once again your goal is the opposite of most traditional businesses, which are attempting to earn profits. You are in the weight *loss* business. You want to produce *losses,* perhaps big *losses.* Remember, in your plan *losses* equate to profits. So you want to have low revenue, or calories in, and high expenses, or calories out, to achieve that loss. That is why you have to allocate calories. I know I am repeating myself, but you have to determine a personal caloric allocation that satisfies you *both* physically and mentally and leads you to success in the weight-loss business.

THE FOOD DIARY

To determine the proper allocation, we will begin by examining your current eating habits. I do not believe one eating program fits all. A program must be customized to each palate and to each lifestyle. When I do my intensive $10,000-a-week plan, I always ask the client to begin a food diary one week prior to my arrival. I request that he or she write everything down, so that I will immediately know when I lay eyes on them if they have been lying. With the diary, I have hard data on their current eating habits and how those habits will need to be modified to fit their new weight-loss plan.

In my thirteen years of experience, very, very few people have lost weight without the food diary. The diary is essential to your success with weight loss. Here is what the Tufts University Health & Nutrition Letter (October 1998) says about writing your food down: "Call it obsessive-compulsive. (The researchers themselves do.) Call it tedious. (It certainly can be.) Even call it a little weird. (It is.) But above all, call it successful. That's because writing down every single thing you eat, along with how many calories it contains, can help you stick to a weight-loss regimen."

KEEPING A FOOD DIARY IS ESSENTIAL TO YOUR SUCCESS

Daniel Kirschenbaum, Ph.D., of Chicago's Center for Behavioral Medicine & Sport Psychology, says keeping a food journal can help people see patterns in their eating. Research shows that those who consistently monitor their food consumption lose weight more steadily and keep it off more successfully than those who don't. That's because the journal keepers can identify the sources of empty calories and know when they resort to overeating.

Interestingly, I have encountered tremendous opposition when I mention the need for a food diary. One woman actually said to me when I suggested a diary, "No way. That is putting way too much emphasis on food." I politely said, "Well, Mrs. X, the choice is yours." What I wanted to say was, "Well, Mrs. X, since you are seventy-five pounds overweight, it would appear that you place a tremendous emphasis on food," but of course I didn't want to risk offending or losing a potential client.

The diary is reality. The diary doesn't lie. The diary contains the data. The diary creates intake awareness. Interestingly, this is a device used by those individuals who want to stop smoking. Smokers are encouraged to write down when they are smoking. This helps to record established patterns and assist smokers in understanding *why* and *when* they are smoking. Understanding this is the same as understanding *why* and *when* you are eating. Once you get past those psychological hurdles, you can then delve into the contents of what you are eating. If you are truly committed to your mission statement, you must employ a food diary and record your eating. This is an essential tool to your success.

Reflect on how often in life we are asked for data. Let's say your division at work misses its quarterly numbers. Your boss calls you in and says, "What was the problem? Show me your numbers." You say, "Oh, I didn't record any numbers. I just thought it would all work out." How long do you think you would be employed?

Or consider the following: Your child's teacher calls your home and tells you that your son or daughter does not take notes in class. You broach the subject, and your child says, "I don't want to take notes. I'll keep all the information [data] in my head. I'll do well on the test." Would you be pleased?

A food diary provides three essential functions. First, as stated in the previous chapter, the diary gives us the "financials" necessary to fill in the first part of our equation, the calories in. Countless people over the years tell me how "good" they have been on their program until I see their diary. The moment I see the data, I can instantly ascertain why they have not lost weight. Once again, this is all about numbers, numbers, numbers.

Here is a great illustration. Many of my clients go out to dinner, frequently to an Italian restaurant, and have two pieces of bread; Caesar salad; pasta with tomato, basil, and olive oil; two glasses of wine; and a few bites of dessert. They smile when they tell me what they ate and look for praise. I look at them and say, "Do you know that was a disaster?"

"What?" they say. "That's my 'healthy' meal. I passed up the lasagna, my favorite!"

Let's examine this "healthy" meal and approximate calories.

Two Pieces of Bread	400 calories
Caesar Salad	650 calories
Tomato, Basil, Olive Oil Pasta	800 calories
Two Glasses of Wine	250 calories
Few Bites of Dessert	200 calories
TOTAL	2,300 CALORIES

You'll notice the "healthy" dinner comes in around 2,300 calories. Obviously, this is not a successful eating plan or caloric allocation. This one meal provides enough calories for the entire day for most individuals. So unless our diners spent the previous part of the day fasting, which is highly unlikely, nor recommended, they have blown their allocation. Briefly note the caloric value of the Caesar salad. Caesar salad dressing is made from olive oil, eggs, Parmesan cheese, and topped with croutons, which are loaded in calories and fat. This salad is a disaster. According to the National Restaurant Association, Caesar salad is the country's most popular main-dish salad and accounts for one-fourth of all salads sold, no doubt in part due to a lack of knowledge on the part of the diner. Most Americans equate salad with light fare and low calories. Did you know most taco salads equal almost 1,000 calories? Clearly, individuals who make these salad choices lack the appropriate level of caloric awareness.

The second purpose of the diary relates to choice. As you walk through your office, kitchen, or the grocery store and you see a small bite of a tasty treat, you pick up the cookie, piece of banana bread, or chocolate, get it really close to your mouth, and think, "If I eat this, I have to go write it down in my diary. Do I? Don't I? Do I? Don't I? Oh, forget it. I'm really not even hungry." Or, you might think, "If I eat this, then I have to cut back drastically at lunch." The diary forces you to make clear choices that simultaneously satisfy your palate and allocate your calories to facilitate weight loss.

Finally, the diary helps you to self-police and create an awareness of what you are eating (calories in). Yes, I know, you would love for someone else to do it for you, but unless you want to ante up $10,000 a week for me to do it, then the job rests on your shoulders and your commitment level to the diary. You might be shocked by the numbers once you input the data. Trust me, it works. Go to my website at *www.businessplanforthebody.com* and download a sample form for the diary. As we established, you are the CEO of this business venture. You would insist on these data from your staff. Why request anything less from yourself?

The following represents a healthy sample diary entry:

TIME	FOOD	PORTION SIZE	CALORIES
8:00 A.M.	Eggs	2 large	180 calories
	Toast	1 slice	80 calories
	Apple	1 medium	100 calories

The Business Plan for the Body

All portion sizes need to be included to the best of your ability. Don't just write chicken breast. Instead, write four, six, or eight ounces of chicken, or use a gauge, such as a deck of cards or the palm of your hand, as a guide. Include all liquid calories, especially water. I know that water does not have any calories, but it is important to record your daily consumption to stay on plan.

So start your food diary today. But how do you assign caloric values to all these foods you are going to be recording? It is relatively easy, but it does require some research to expand your current knowledge of caloric awareness.

ACQUIRE CALORIC AWARENESS

Caloric awareness is simply understanding and knowing the caloric value of foods and the appropriate portion size. You can purchase any number of books detailing the caloric value of most foods, such as *Corinne Netzer's Complete Book of Food Counts,* or surf the Internet at *www.nutri-facts.com/main.asp,* which will allow you to plug in the foods, and the website will do the calculation for free. You need to know the values, which includes the calories per serving and portion size.

Take olive oil as an example. Few people are aware of the caloric and fat content of olive oil. The media have devoted a great deal of space in recent years to Mediterranean menus that incorporate olive oil and have extolled its healthy benefits. Olive oil does not have cholesterol, but it is 100 percent fat, packs 120 calo-   **CALORIES**
ries per tablespoon, and has approximately 13.3   **DO COUNT**
grams of fat. Putting three tablespoons of olive oil on food is the equivalent of three, four-ounce scoops of ice cream. Not exactly what I would call a "healthy" food.

Now, if you compare olive oil to coconut, palm, or numerous other oils that are loaded in fat *and* cholesterol, then I would agree olive oil is a better choice, but come on. Manslaughter carries a lighter sentence than murder one, but bottom line, the victim is still dead. Same applies to olive oil. Anything that is 100 percent fat and 120 calories a tablespoon does not constitute a wise choice for an individual who desires to lose or keep weight off, unless it is used sparingly. Also, keep in mind that Mediterranean portions and North American portions vary tremendously. I'm Greek, raised by Greeks, and I've been to Greece numerous times. Mediterraneans eat tons of fruit, vegetables, little meat, and yes, they use olive

DON'T SUFFER FROM PORTION DISTORTION

oil. They also eat *small* portions. North Americans demand and consume *enormous* portions. I have gone to numerous Greek restaurants across the country. The American portion size compared to a true Mediterranean portion size is huge, probably about two and one-half times as large. Remember, large portions translate into large caloric intake, whether the food is Greek, American, Italian, Indian, Cajun, Mexican, Chinese, or any number of others.

According to researchers at New York University, "Fat or skinny, human beings are appallingly bad at estimating portion sizes. And the larger the portion size, the less accurate we get."

So that is your next assignment. Simultaneously, start a food diary *and* do research on the caloric value of foods. Numerous studies indicate that overweight subjects low-ball their calorie intake by one-half. I totally agree with this, as my experience discussing caloric intake with clients has indicated that they possess very little awareness of the amount of food they are eating and the caloric content of that food.

FAT CONTENT IN FOODS

At this point you are probably asking yourself, "But what about the fat content of various foods?" You will hear me say this over and over again: The calorie counts much more in the weight-loss business than the fat content. A recent statistic revealed that 50 percent say their biggest diet concern is how much fat they eat. Do you know what percentage said *calories* were their biggest concern? Only 8 percent. This is a tremendous error in judgment and one of the top five reasons why we have gotten so overweight. Granted, fat has gotten all the press and has been deemed the villain when it comes to Americans' weight gain. But I believe we have all been somewhat duped. Go back to Chapter 2 and my discussion of Fallacy 4, "I am eating fat-free or low-fat." That will answer many of your ques-

The Business Plan for the Body

tions. Fat is not the culprit. Overeating is. If I could give you just one piece of advice on how to lose weight successfully, it would be: *count the calories.*

CALORIC DENSITY

Caloric density is commonly defined as a food's calories divided by its weight. A recent study by Susan Roberts, of the Jean Mayer U.S. Department of Agriculture Human Nutrition Research Center on Aging at Tufts University, showed that "it's calorie density, not fat, that determines how many calories people eat." A colleague of Susan Roberts, Megan McCrory, continues with, "Fat is important to watch out for, but low-fat foods that are high in sugar, like SnackWell's cookies and Entenmann's cakes, are also high in caloric density." Both Roberts and McCrory conclude, "Fruits, vegetables, and other high-fiber foods can keep weight off, calorie-dense foods do not."

Once again, this is where the bread, pasta, bagels, and fat-free snacks—such as cookies, cakes, and chips—are commonly misunderstood. There is nothing wrong with these foods. What is wrong is the average American's overconsumption of these foods with the belief that they will not cause them to gain weight. These foods all have a high caloric density, therefore, bite for bite, an individual is consuming a great deal of calories.

"The most startling aspect of the weight difference between Americans and Europeans is that, according to the advice regularly doled out by American experts and according to the accepted American wisdom, the Europeans are doing everything wrong. Many of their stores do not sell skim milk. Low and non-fat desserts are almost nonexistent in Europe. They haven't the least idea what a SnackWell's is." This observation of Michael Fumento, author of *The Fat of the Land: the Obesity Epidemic and How Overweight Americans Can Help Themselves,* once again illustrates Americans' belief that fat-free equates to calorie-free. This is not the case.

A few additional rules regarding the food diary. One, keep the diary with you at all times. Put it in your purse, briefcase, breast pocket, Palm Pilot, or personal organizer. Look, none of us is traveling light. We make room for keys, wallets, money clips, daily planners, makeup, portable phones, digital diaries, and ChapStick. We can all make room for a two-by-four-inch, two-ounce diary. Rule two, record soon after you eat. None of this "I'll do it at the end of each day." Fill it in immediately after eating so you have a written and mental note of what you have consumed each day. As you will see in the following chapters, you will be asked to record data on your exercise program and body weight as well as your eating. This one journal will then contain your entire eating and exercise program as well as documenting your progress. Some of you might want to transfer these data on a daily basis to your home or office computer.

Don't forget, you "went public." You should not be hiding in a corner, shielding your diary like a criminal as you make your eating entries. Pull the diary out after a meal with confidence.

FOOD DIARIES NEVER LIE

Finally, rule three, *all* food consumed must be written down. Entries such as "bad lunch" do not exist. You must be specific. Write down the foods and liquids consumed during the "bad lunch" and plug in those caloric values. You will quickly learn that some items previously thought to be "bad" are not so bad and some "bad" are truly a disaster. Diaries provide a realistic picture of where you need to make adjustments. Diaries can also help you identify situations or states of mind that trigger overeating. Many long-term weight losers use food diaries as a tool to get back on track when the pounds start creeping up. Bottom line, a food diary is a reflection of your behavior. It provides you with a clear picture of what you are consuming.

I have been on my own weight control program for almost two decades. I no longer keep a written food diary, but I keep a mental diary every day and know what I have consumed. So don't think you will be bound to this written diary for life. This is a tool to success; use it as such. If you are losing weight and keeping the weight off, hey, you're in the weight-loss business. If you then feel you can eliminate the diary, try it. If you start gaining weight, get it back out. Period. But remember, it's wise to always keep a mental food diary of what you are consuming throughout each day.

The Business Plan for the Body

WHAT TO EAT AND WHY

In the previous chapter, you filled in the basal metabolic rate equation and the activity multiplier. You determined the calories your body requires on a daily basis. Once you have established that number, we can proceed to devise a food program compatible with your personal palate, and one that facilitates weight loss. What foods satisfy you? Everyone has a personal list of likes and dislikes. I am often confronted by people who say, "I hate celery and carrots. I won't eat them." Fine, who said that a weight-loss eating program requires celery and carrots? What it does require is the proper balance of foods that physically and mentally satisfy your needs.

For most people, eating is 20 percent physical and 80 percent emotional. As Americans, we eat when we are happy, sad, celebrating, consoling, in love and out of love. We use food all the time. Something everyone needs to do is to examine their emotional relationship with food. According to Michael R. Lowe, Ph.D., a professor in the Department of Clinical and Health Psychology at MCP Hahnemann University in Philadelphia, "There are many reasons why we overindulge, but the habit generally follows one of three typical patterns. One, you simply unconsciously take in more calories a day. Two, you knowingly eat more than you should. And three, binge eating, where you take in considerable amounts of food and feel totally out of control when you are doing it." You need to determine into which category you fall.

EXAMINE YOUR EMOTIONAL RELATIONSHIP WITH FOOD

In my experience, very few people fall into category one, and don't realize that they are taking in more calories than they are expending. Rather, they attribute the weight gain not to their eating but to the erroneous factors we have already discussed, such as bad genes or slow metabolism. The majority of people I have dealt with fall into category two, and knowingly eat too much but have difficulty controlling their eating and maintaining a consistent exercise program. The third group, the binge eaters, definitely have the most difficult challenge, since this pattern of eating is connected to deep psychological issues that are temporarily masked, or briefly soothed, as they consume huge amounts of calories. Some binge eaters consume thousands of calories in one very brief sitting. Experts say we crave carbohydrates because they stimulate production of serotonin (a brain chemical that regulates mood and sleepiness and seems to calm anxiety and induce relaxation). Interestingly, most popular antidepressant drugs such as Prozac, Zoloft, and the like are all serotonin enhancers. So, by eating foods that stimulate the production of serotonin, in essence you are self-medicating.

Okay, you are now aware that weight loss is determined by the following equation: calories in minus calories out. And your goal is to produce big weight losses. You simultaneously begin a food diary and improve your caloric awareness. As you begin developing your customized weight-loss eating allocation, here are some parameters I want you to follow.

EATING ALLOCATION PARAMETERS

YOU MUST EAT A MINIMUM OF FIVE SERVINGS OF VEGETABLES EACH DAY

Vegetables are packed with vitamins and minerals, loaded with water and fiber, and they are low in calories. A cup of cut veggies, or one serving, contains approximately 35 to 50 calories. Eat as many types as you can, since each vegetable supplies different essential nutrients.

I am repeatedly asked: Do the vegetables have to be fresh? The answer is no. The University of Illinois Department of Food Science and Human Nutrition conducted a study analyzing the nutritive values of fourteen different fresh, canned, and frozen fruits and vegetables. The results confirmed that, in most cases, canned or frozen fruits and vegetables are nutritionally comparable to their prepared fresh counterparts.

DON'T WORRY ABOUT FRESH VS. FROZEN VEGETABLES

The key to freshness in a vegetable is the harvesting process. If a vegetable is picked at the optimum time, immediately frozen, and then placed in distribution channels, it will retain most of its vitamins and nutrients. If the same vegetable, not picked at peak time, sat for a while before freezing, then many of its vitamins and nutrients will have diminished. The same applies to a vegetable that is sold fresh. A fresh vegetable that is picked, immediately delivered to the store, sold, and eaten will also retain the majority of its nutrients and vitamins. The same fresh vegetable hangs out in the store too long? I think you get the pattern. When you shop for fresh vegetables, really take a moment to select the best quality. This unfortunately is one of the pitfalls of on-line shopping, or a shopping service where someone other than you does the picking. Don't be concerned about the fresh versus frozen argument. Just make it as easy for yourself as possible. If that means loading your freezer with frozen vegetables, fine. If your palate prefers the fresh, fine. Just eat them.

The USDA's Agricultural Research Service completed a study on Americans' eating habits in 1994 that revealed that most Americans are eating only three servings, or three cups, of vegetables a day, and 40 percent of those servings are coming from french fries and mashed potatoes! Think about it, mashed potatoes and french fries! Now, I am not opposed to potatoes, which are very healthy and packed with nutrients and vitamins. What I am opposed to is the deep frying and the added cream, butter, sour cream, cheese, bacon bits, and other high-calorie ingredients that Americans like to dump on their potatoes. Consequently, the chances are great that you and most Americans are not close to my recommendation of five servings of vegetables a day. Where are the dark green leafy vegetables? Don't even think of counting fries or ketchup as a vegetable. Instead, think spinach, asparagus, broccoli, and sweet potato (which most nutritionists agree is the single most nutritious food you can eat because it is loaded with vitamins and minerals); green, red, and yellow peppers (the second most nutritious foods you can eat); mushrooms, tomatoes, and carrots.

THE BRIGHTER THE COLOR, THE MORE NUTRIENTS AND VITAMINS

YOU MUST INCLUDE THREE SERVINGS OF FRUIT EACH DAY

Like vegetables, fruit is packed with vitamins and nutrients, filled with water and fiber, and supply between 50 to 100 calories for a medium-size piece, or one cup, cut up (which equals one serving). Fruit makes a great dessert because it's a tasty, low-calorie way to satisfy a sweet craving. The same research conducted in 1994 by the USDA showed that only 24 percent of Americans are eating two servings of fruit a day, and that occurs only because they are including fruit such as the apples in apple pie and the fruit filling in a Danish. Not impressive. Don't even think of including a Pop-Tart or jelly doughnut as your fruit.

Some interesting research from New Zealand's University of Auckland revealed that the weight of food may be more important than fat and calories when it comes to weight loss. Individuals tend to eat the same weight of food each day. What foods weigh the most with the least amount of calories? Fruits and vegetables, whose high water and fiber content keep them high in weight. A navel orange, for instance, weighs two and a half times as much as a croissant but contains approximately 60 calories. The croissant can be hundreds of calories but weighs very little. Light foods such as popcorn, cheese puffs, rice cakes, and Twinkies don't weigh very much but have lots of calories. Consider the weight of the food you are eating and realize that the heavier items are often lower in calories.

Why have I been so emphatic about eating vegetables and fruit? Because they fill you up and are enormously healthy. Vegetables and fruit are low in calories and, once again, are loaded with vitamins, minerals, fiber, and water. Think of eating vegetables and fruit as your core curriculum. Reach for fruits and vegetables instead of other snacks, and minimize your caloric intake. Trust me, eat my recommended servings and you will be on your way to success in the weight-loss business.

IT IS IMPERATIVE TO EAT A SMALL AMOUNT OF PROTEIN WITH EACH MEAL

My definition of protein includes egg whites, yogurt, cottage cheese, boneless, skinless chicken breast, white meat turkey, fish, seafood (shrimp, as well as other shellfish), along with other lean meats and legumes. Protein is the most difficult food for your body to digest. Therefore, eating protein with each meal will keep you physically full longer. Once again, I am not advocating a high-protein diet. I am advocating a diet that includes a *small* amount (approximately a cup of yogurt or cottage cheese, four to eight ounces of animal protein or egg whites) with every meal.

The Business Plan for the Body

PLAN A FEW SMALL SNACKS DURING THE DAY, SPECIFICALLY IN THE LATE MORNING, LATE AFTERNOON, AND AFTER DINNER

Numerous studies show that when people leave too much time in between meals, they will overeat at the next meal. If you eat breakfast at 6:30 A.M. and do not plan on lunch until 1:00 P.M., chances are that you will be starving. This is the type of schedule that can lead to overeating and straying from the plan. Think about it: You're hungry, the bread basket comes, and you dive in. I would. Or you walk through your office or kitchen and grab a few handfuls of something because you're starving. But what if around 10:30 A.M. you ate a piece of fruit, a 100-calorie yogurt, or some turkey slices (these are all my personal favorites). When lunch comes along, you won't be starving. Again, work the numbers. Eat a 100-calorie snack and skip eating 400 to 500 calories of bread or munchies before lunch. What happens? You start to lose weight.

EAT A 100-CALORIE SNACK TO PREVENT A 1,000-CALORIE BINGE

DON'T FEEL GUILTY ABOUT HIGH-FAT, HIGH-CALORIE TREATS

If you love chocolate, then allocate a few hundred calories each day. I personally love Gummy Bears, licorice, and other "chewy" candies. Many days I eat some, but I know the calorie count. I actually walk into a drugstore, buy two large Gummy Bears for a total of 100 calories (they are 50 calories each) and eat them. Mind you, I don't buy a bag and tell myself I am only going to eat a few. No way. I know that if they are in my possession, I will eat them. Ditto with baked potato chips. I love baked potato chips, but I never buy the big bag. I buy the single serving, a 120-calorie bag, and dive in. If I bought the larger size, I know I would polish off the bag. So I allocate, but I also minimize the risk of overeating by purchasing and possessing only a small portion.

NO FOOD IS A "NO" IF YOU KNOW THE NUMBERS

Of course, I realize that buying the small bags is more expensive. If you are careful with your money, as I urge you to be, then buy the big bag, but split it up in individual plastic bags so you know your portion size and can assign calories. This way you won't open the bag and estimate.

No food should be a "no." You simply have to know the calorie count and how to control your portion size. Saying "no" to a food or food group will most likely lead to a binge. If you love bread, then find a 50- or 60-calorie-a-slice bread and enjoy. If you love red meat, then find a lean cut, eat four to six ounces, and enjoy. Again, this is your body, and only you know what foods physically and mentally satisfy your needs. This is why I don't give you a set eating program to follow. Let me use myself as an illustration. Keep in mind that what works for me (and the number we determined in Chapter 5 for my daily caloric needs) may or may not work for you. This is what I frequently do to stay on plan.

JIM KARAS' TYPICAL FOOD DIARY ENTRY

Before My Workout	One Piece of Fruit	100 calories
Breakfast	Two Pieces of 60-Calorie Bread	120 calories
	Sliced Turkey	150 calories
	Sliced Tomato	50 calories
	One Serving of Fruit	100 calories
Snack	One Fat-Free Yogurt	100 calories
Lunch	Egg White Omelette in Nonstick Spray with Spinach and Tomato	200 calories
	Grilled Potatoes in Nonstick Spray	200 calories
	Tomato Salad with Balsamic Vinegar	200 calories
Snack	Gummy Candy	100 calories
	One Serving of Fruit	100 calories
Dinner	Grilled Chicken	400 calories
	Huge Salad with Lettuce, Tomato, Carrots, Mushrooms, etc.	300 calories
	Steamed Vegetables	200 calories
	8 Ounces of Wine	200 calories
Snack	Portion of Low-Fat Frozen Yogurt or Pretzel Cookies	200 calories
	TOTAL	2,720 calories

You may notice that my calories are heavily weighted at dinner. That is my life. Whether it be with family or friends, dinner is the time I consume the greatest amount of my daily calories. This does not mean that I overeat. I stay within my allotment for the day. Clearly, when I go out to dinner, I probably eat more calories, since, as much as I try, the preparation of my food is not within my control. But I am realistic. This style of eating keeps me at the weight I desire.

Once again, this is all part of your information-gathering stage. You need to sit down and study the caloric values of your

The Business Plan for the Body

favorite foods. If you eat fast food frequently, then buy a book that gives the caloric values of most fast foods, or go to the Internet at *http://www.kenkuhl.com/fastfood/* or *www.dietriot.com/fff/*. McDonald's is now displaying a chart that shows the caloric, fat, and sodium values of its foods. Always know your numbers, and if you don't, then conservatively estimate until you get the necessary data. You are creating caloric awareness.

YOU CAN EAT FAST FOOD AND BE ON PLAN

The following chart lists some of the best and worst fast-food choices:

THE BEST AND WORST OF FAST FOOD

RESTAURANT	FOOD	CALORIES	FAT GRAMS	SODIUM
McDonald's				
	Grilled Chicken Salad with Fat-Free Dressing	150	1	240
	Hamburger	270	9	600
	Small Fries	210	10	135
	Big Xtra with Cheese	810	55	1,870
	Super Size Fries	610	29	390
Burger King				
	Hamburger	320	15	520
	Small Fries	250	13	550
	Double Whopper w/Cheese	1,010	67	1,460
	King Size Fries	590	30	1,110
Subway				
	6-Inch Roast Beef Sub	296	5	928
	6-Inch Super Italian Sub	668	39	2,576
Taco Bell				
	Chili Cheese Burrito	330	13	900
	Taco Salad with Salsa	850	52	2,250
Wendy's				
	Grilled Chicken Sandwich	310	8	790
	Big Bacon Classic	580	30	1,460

As illustrated, fast food can be low in calories if you make the correct selections or choices. However, observe the following example. A traditional McDonald's burger and a small order of fries is approximately 480 calories and 19 grams of fat. Switch to a Big Xtra with cheese and a large fries and your meal packs 1,420 calories and 84 grams of fat. A disaster. Once again, the responsibility and the caloric choice rests with you. Yes, you can eat fast food and be on plan.

VISUALIZE
PROPER
PORTION
SIZE

As mentioned in Chapter 2, it's all numbers. All the frenzy surrounding high-protein, low-carbohydrate diets has to do with calories. Again, it's all numbers. Lots of bread, pasta, and fat-free treats are low in fat, but very high in calories. There is nothing wrong with bread and pasta. What is wrong is the American perception of portion size. France and Italy, two countries revered for their world-class cuisines, have a far smaller percentage of overweight citizens than North America. The American perception of the size of Italians and the true size of Italians is vastly different. Our perception of Italians is Mama Celeste, Luciano Pavarotti, or some of the cast members of *The Sopranos*. In reality, Italians are thin (think Sophia Loren). They can fit into all that little Armani and Prada clothing because they consume portion-controlled amounts. Eating Italian or French cuisine doesn't make Italians or the French fat. It's Americans eating Italian and French food with no portion control that creates overweight Americans.

SIZE MATTERS

The problem is not the food, it's the portion size. America is the land of the thirty-two-ounce Porterhouse steak. Lobster, a harmless shellfish, has to be dipped in drawn butter. Most salad bars present you with a plate the size of a serving platter and are nothing more than the resting place of fatty meat, cheese, mayonnaise, and creamy salad dressing. If you want to eat 400 calories of pasta, go ahead, just know that 400 calories of pasta is not a great deal of food (remember our discussion of caloric density). Try this test. Buy an inexpensive one pound box of pasta. The average box is 1,600 calories in total. Now boil all the pasta and look at the cooked portion. That is 1,600 calories.

The Business Plan for the Body

Separate in half, that is 800 calories. Cut it in half again, that is 400 calories. Cut it one more time, that is 200 calories. Now, tell me, honestly, which is your "normal" portion size? Probably at the high end. By the way, please refrigerate this cooked pasta in a container and don't feel, since you completed this test, compelled to eat it. Mind you, this is *before* the sauce, which generally is loaded with calories and fat. Also, know that most restaurants coat the pasta noodles with oil, butter, or another fat before they even put on the sauce to prevent the pasta from sticking. So you end up with high-calorie, low-fat pasta noodles, tossed in oil, butter, or other fats, *before* you add the sauce. This all translates into huge caloric numbers. Pasta should be a side dish, eaten in *small* portions, whereas Americans eat huge portions of everything on a daily basis. In Italy, pasta comes as a small course before the entrée. The portion size amounts to about four twirls of a fork. Now think about your average twirl.

TAKE THE SERVING-SIZE CHALLENGE

Same applies to bread. Do you realize that most retail bagels are over 500 calories each, and that is before one applies cream cheese or other toppings? Big numbers. A recent study asked a hundred college students to find a "medium"-size bagel, baked potato, muffin, apple, or cookie. The items the students brought back were as much as three times larger than the amounts defined as standard serving sizes by the USDA's food pyramid. Clearly, this illustrates that Americans suffer from a severe case of portion and size distortion.

Here are some additional methods to help you visualize proper portion size: one cup of rice, vegetables, fruit, etc., is approximately the size of an average fist; three ounces of meat, fish, or poultry, approximately the size of your palm or a deck of cards; your thumb tip represents a teaspoon, three thumb tips equal a tablespoon; one medium apple or orange, the size of a baseball; one ounce of cheese, the size of four dice. Remember, keep eyeballing your food to keep a handle on portion size. But most of all, buy a measuring cup and a food scale. They will really make a difference when it comes to your caloric education. You don't have to use them forever, just long enough to get a feel for the portion size and the corresponding caloric value. You will find that you learn these values very quickly.

READ LABELS

Fortunately, most manufacturers are required by law to list the amount of calories, fat content, carbohydrate, sodium, etc., on most of their products. The data are there in black and white. Again, the choice is yours. You would be amazed how many clients have called me over the years and said things like, "I just read the label on my favorite can of soup and I was shocked." This kind of surprise happens all the time, so read the labels. Researchers at the Fred Hutchinson Cancer Center have found that people who read labels eat less than those who don't.

The most important data from the label include the calories per serving or portion, the portion size, and the number of portions per container. Look at Entenmann's Fat-Free Cakes. Many of them are 110 to 120 calories a serving. Then look at the fact that there are ten servings per cake. That would make each serving very, very small. You probably eat four or five servings, deluding yourself into believing that it was one, maybe one and a half, servings. Remember what I urged you to do with a box of pasta. Once you see the reality of the portion size, you will understand the reality of the numbers.

See the sample label on page 101. When you look at a food label, please observe the following:

1. Look at the serving size. In the sample label, the serving size is one-half cup. If necessary, get out a measuring cup and fill it up. That is the serving size.

2. Look at the servings per package or container. In this example, there are four. Just as I used the example of the Entenmann's cake, notice how many total servings there are in the package or container. Remember this number when you look at calories per serving.

3. Look at the calories per serving. This is the amount of calories in the serving size you have identified. In our example, there are four servings of 260 calories. Multiply the number of servings and you will arrive at the total number of calories for the entire package or container. In our example, that would be 1040 calories. Now, be honest. What portion do you normally consume?

Get out your favorite ice cream or frozen yogurt bowl and fill it with your average portion. Take that portion out and measure it in a measuring cup. That will give you a clearer indication of the number of calories you are consuming. Are you eating only one portion? Probably not.

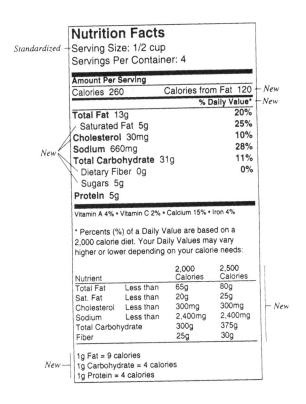

There are additional data on a food label, such as the calories from fat and the quantity of saturated fat, sodium, carbohydrate, fiber, and protein. The label also lists daily percentage values of certain vitamins. While these data are valuable, right now I want you to focus on the serving size and the caloric value to properly allocate your calories.

Beware of variety. Numerous case studies have shown that the more selections presented to an individual, such as at a buffet or passed hors d'oeuvres (remember this chapter's opening anecdote), the more he or she will eat. The American Dietetic Association and other health organizations encourage Americans to eat a variety of foods, a practice I

TOO MUCH VARIETY CAN ENCOURAGE OVEREATING

endorse. But by variety the ADA is advocating the inclusion of a variety of fruits and vegetables into one's diet, because they are packed with different vitamins and nutrients and are low in calories. When is variety to be avoided? When you are presented with numerous choices at one time (again, the large buffet, platters of hors d'oeuvres). According to Megan McCrory of Tufts University, "If people are offered three different kinds of sandwiches, they'll eat more than if they are given three of the same. People eat more pasta if they have three shapes to choose from, even if all three are the same color and served with the same sauce." So what is the message? Be careful with variety. Exercise caution when invited to a buffet brunch or when hors d'oeuvres are served. Think before you eat. But variety is always okay as long as it consists of fruits and vegetables.

WHAT ABOUT LIQUID CALORIES?

Water is the single most important beverage for you to drink. Water has no calories. I am a huge water drinker. Currently, most health organizations claim Americans should drink eight, eight-ounce glasses of water each day. But look at how vague that recommendation is. Say you are a young man, an athlete, six feet tall, 175 pounds, and play basketball five times a week for a few hours. How can 64 ounces of water each day even come close to your body's needs? Do you live in a very dry climate, such as the desert, or at high altitude? Do you take medication? Are you pregnant or ill? Or are you getting older and don't feel thirst as readily? In each of these situations, your body will require more water.

EIGHT GLASSES OF WATER MAY NOT BE ENOUGH

Each and every person generally needs much more than sixty-four ounces a day. Consider that your total body weight is almost three-quarters water and that water is necessary for all chemical reactions in the body. No wonder people can survive for weeks without food, but only a few days without fluids. In addition, water can:

- Reduce the risk of cancer. *Water speeds the elimination of fecal matter from the colon and urine from the bladder, reducing both colon and bladder cancer, respectively. By decreas-*

The Business Plan for the Body

ing the amount of time waste matter remains in the body, one reduces the risk of potential carcinogens in the system.

- Decrease the frequency of asthma attacks. *Researchers have documented the relationship between dehydration and asthma attacks.*
- Diminish the risk of kidney stones. *Consumption of water prevents the formation of crystals from calcium, uric acid, and other substances.*
- Improve oral health and breath. *Many oral problems are attributable to dehydration. Saliva, which is enhanced by proper hydration, neutralizes cavity-causing acids in the mouth. Drinking water also washes away food particles and sugars and inhibits the growth of microorganisms that contribute to oral problems such as gum disease.*
- Assist seniors to cope with dehydration. *Dehydration is one of the top ten reasons why older people are hospitalized. After the average individual is "down" by approximately thirty-two ounces of water, most thirst mechanisms kick in. But as we age, this mechanism begins to falter. Therefore, the elderly must be that much more aware of their water consumption and consume water even when they are not thirsty.*

What about water and weight loss? According to Dr. Donald Robertson, medical director of the Southwest Bariatric Nutrition Center in Scottsdale, Arizona, "If people who are trying to lose weight don't drink enough water, the body can't metabolize the fat adequately." Therefore, weight loss will occur more efficiently in a properly hydrated environment. Plus, drinking water may help curb appetite and make you feel fuller, and some people simply confuse thirst with hunger. Clearly, drinking more water enhances your health, appearance, and ability to lose weight. So take a break, put this book down, and go fill a nice tall glass with water and drink. You just made an intelligent, well-researched decision in the weight-loss business.

Can food improve your water balance? Certainly. Most fruits and vegetables are high water content foods, so eat up.

When you begin to drink more water, you will find that you have to urinate more frequently. I have clients who shop on Michigan Avenue, Madison Avenue, and Rodeo Drive, who have become

WATER
HELPS TO
METABOLIZE
FAT

experts on the location of public rest rooms along these streets. But after the first few weeks, your body will adjust so that you have to go to the bathroom less frequently, but with greater volume. Just give it some time. And remember, it is a small, small price to pay for better health. I will go so far as to say that if you decide to reject my plan for weight loss and improved health, but do decide to drink more water, I would still feel a sense of accomplishment.

What about other liquids? Let's start with coffee, tea, or diet soda. Do these improve or diminish your water balance? That depends on whether they contain caffeine. If they are caffeine-free, then they do count toward your water balance. If they are caffeinated, then they do not count, as they are diuretics and boost urine output, which could leave you even more dehydrated.

I discuss alcohol and its effects on the body in Chapter 9, but briefly, alcohol is very dehydrating, since it robs the body of water as it is broken down by the body. In fact, if you consume alcohol, you should consume additional water. Alcohol should never count toward daily water intake.

Soup? That clearly depends on the amount of sodium in the soup. Soup does contain water, but that water is canceled out by the amount of sodium. Most soups served in restaurants contain over 2,500 milligrams of sodium, which is more than the daily recommended amount. So, just say no to soup when it comes to water balance. Also, soup is generally loaded in calories, so I urge my clients to avoid it entirely. The exception is homemade or labeled soup so you know the calorie count.

Allow me to elaborate on this for a moment. You go to lunch. You are trying to lose weight. You order soup and salad. Unless you know for sure that it was prepared in a low-fat manner, the soup, even though it is just chicken soup, is high in fat, sodium, and calories. The salad has dressing on it. Your "healthy" lunch could be well over 1,000 calories. Your weight-loss venture goes bust.

In addition, a recent study at Purdue University identified an important distinction between calories derived from liquid and calories derived from solid food. Nutritionist Dr. Richard Mattes gave one group of individuals 400 calories of jelly beans a day and the other 400 calories of soda pop. What he identified was that the jelly bean group ate less food throughout the day, so that the body properly accounted for the fact that 400 additional calories were being consumed. On the other hand, the

The Business Plan for the Body

soda group ate just as much as always and did not compensate for the fact that 400 additional calories of a liquid had been consumed. "A particular problem with fluid calories," Dr. Mattes says, "is that they don't tip satiety mechanisms as effectively as solid foods."

The lesson to be learned: Stop drinking your calories, and that includes juice, soda, alcohol (which can also depress your metabolism—see Chapter 9), so-called performance drinks (which are mostly a marketing sham and are loaded with sugar), lattes, cappuccinos, and similar drinks, unless they are in moderation and you are aware of their caloric content. As an alternative, order an espresso drink prepared with nonfat milk, which steams or froths up perfectly. Most juice is 15 calories an ounce; wine, 25 calories an ounce. My four-year-old daughter drinks tiny juice boxes pierced with a straw all the time. Do you know that they are 90 calories each? Huge numbers for that amount of liquid. For most children, this is too many calories. Don't forget, childhood obesity is at the highest level in our history. Most parents are thrilled when they tell me that "Johnny" doesn't drink soda pop but instead drinks juice or Gatorade. That is a disaster. There is little difference calorically between soda, juice, and Gatorade. They are all loaded with calories. And forget smoothies. Many homemade or purchased smoothies can pack 500 calories in one serving, because they are made with double portions of frozen yogurt (or regular yogurt) and are a lot bigger than one cup. Think about it. You work out for an hour, sweat, shower, change, then negate the calories you burned in one "healthy" smoothie. Not smart, unless you know exactly what's going into the blender and can control the calories yourself.

So what is the message? Think before you drink. If you want to include liquid calories, as I do when I drink wine, be aware of the portion size and the associated caloric value. The same applies to a cocktail.

LIQUID CALORIES DON'T TRIGGER SATIATION LEVELS

STRATEGIC ACTION PLAN

- *You have learned that weight loss is achieved by numbers.*
- *Numbers must be inserted into the following equation:* calories in minus calories out = body weight.

- *A food diary is imperative. In it, you will record all food items in the order in which they were consumed. Do not omit your liquid consumption.*
- *Record in your food diary immediately after consumption.*
- *Eat five servings of vegetables and three servings of fruit every day.*
- *Include a small amount of protein with each meal.*
- *You may plan each day to include a late morning, late afternoon, or after-dinner snack as it fits into your caloric allocation.*
- *Eat foods that mentally as well as physically satisfy you. In other words, nothing is a "no," but you must be aware of and allocate those calories. Again, remember, this is a program based on numbers.*
- *Be aware of portion size and accordingly exercise portion control. No longer suffer from portion distortion.*
- *Be aware of the caloric value of everything you put in your mouth, and strive to improve your "caloric awareness."*
- *Drink lots and lots of water and consume foods with a high water content, such as fruits and vegetables.*
- *Refrain from drinking high-calorie beverages, such as sugary soda and juice. Remember, liquid calories do not trigger satiety mechanisms the way solid food does.*
- *Exposure to a variety of different foods, such as at a buffet or hors d'oeuvres, can cause overeating. Be very careful in those situations.*
- *You will behave intelligently. You will stay on plan.*

Begin your program today. Don't wait until January 1, an upcoming wedding, your twenty-fifth high school reunion, or a Monday. I always used to begin a crazy new diet on Mondays thinking it would be a fresh start. I even fasted for about three years every Monday as a way to control my weight, which was ridiculous. All I really ended up doing was overeating on Sunday in anticipation of the fast *and* overeating on Tuesday since I was starving. Not an intelligent weight-loss strategy. All that you are doing by waiting until an "official" starting date is procrastinating.

You have the power to change many things about your present life. So become a little trendy. Join the empowerment movement. Take control of what you put in your mouth.

Remember, you are creating a business plan for your body. The essential component of that plan is the following equation:

Calories In – Calories out = Body Weight

You now possess the tools to successfully manipulate and allocate the first part of this equation, the calories in. Now on to Chapter 7 for information on maximizing the second part of the equation, the calories out.

PRESERVATION OF CAPITAL

7

Keeping Your Muscle

Go to any health club. Walk into the cardio-vascular room. What do you see? Dozens, maybe hundreds, of people on treadmills, StairMasters, bikes, elliptical trainers, or other assorted cardiovascular equipment. Notice that the vast majority of these individuals are over-weight. Many of these people spend hours each week on one of these machines or a combination thereof, desperate to lose weight, and firmly believing that all this cardiovascular exercise will burn hundreds, even thousands, of calories and enable them to achieve their goal, weight loss.

Now, go to the strength and resistance room. What do you see? The majority of individuals doing strength and resistance exercises are in vastly better shape. In which room should you spend the majority of your time?

As we know from investing, whether it be in real estate or the stock or bond market, one of the key considerations of any investment is preservation of capital. We know that first and foremost we want to keep that capital—in other words, not lose money—and derive a profit from the investment. This same approach needs to be applied to your exercise plan. You want to derive a profit from your program.

When I meet a potential new client, one of my first questions is: "Why do you want to exercise?" I am often astounded by the number

> **"I find that the harder I work, the more luck I seem to have."**
>
> THOMAS JEFFERSON

of people who look at me and say, "I don't know, aren't you supposed to?" Yes, of course you are supposed to exercise. I will go so far as to say that exercise is the equivalent of the Fountain of Youth. But the fact remains, most people have no idea why they should exercise and what type of exercise to do.

Scientists say physical activity is the single biggest predictor of who successfully keeps the pounds off and who puts them right back on. Yet approximately 60 percent of American adults perform little or no physical activity.

MUSCLE IS YOUR CAPITAL— PRESERVE IT

If your goal is weight loss—and I assume for the majority of you it is—then you should exercise for this basic reason: the preservation of muscle. In *The Business Plan for the Body*, muscle is your "capital." We know from Chapters 2 and 6 that muscle is the most metabolically active tissue in the body, which will in turn increase your basal metabolic rate and enable you to burn more calories twenty-four hours a day.

The Principal Reason to Exercise

The principal reason to exercise should be to preserve and increase lean muscle tissue, which can only be accomplished through strength and resistance exercises. The more you preserve and increase lean muscle tissue, the more you will increase "expenses," or calories out, in your weight-loss equation. Remember, your goal is losses, so the more you *expend*, the more weight you will lose.

Once again we are flipping the classic business terminology. Most businesses are established to create profits. Our business is being created to produce losses. Your weight *loss* is your profit.

Strength and resistance training is the key to weight loss. As we know, one pound of additional lean muscle tissue can burn from 35 to 50 calories per day. Remember, five pounds of additional lean muscle tissue can burn 91,250 calories a year, which is the equivalent of more than twenty-six pounds of body fat lost annually. That number is significant. But you're thinking, "I bet I have to kill myself to add this much lean muscle tissue." Absolutely not. On the contrary, adding lean muscle is easier than you think. All you need is a plan.

WEIGHT LOSS IS YOUR PROFIT

This plan is called an *exercise prescription*. Think of being overweight and out of shape as an illness. If you are sick, you call or go to the doctor and describe your symptoms. Given those symptoms and possibly other

tests, the doctor will write a prescription, including the medication, strength, and dosage. If you are not better in time, the doctor may adjust or change that prescription. How many of you have considered being overweight and out of shape an illness? It's time to think of it that way. What I am advocating is the creation and utilization of an exercise prescription to specifically treat this illness.

The same applies to a business. Over the course of time, many organizations lose sight of their original mission. In the 1980s numerous conglomerates were formed by combining various companies that provided little if any business synergy. It didn't work. They drifted from their core product or service. (Remember the New Coke, or United Airlines branching into the car rental and hotel business and briefly changing its name to Allegis?) In other words, they strayed from their plan. Frequently, outside consultants are called upon to shape and refocus the organization. They provide a new strategic plan; in other words, a new prescription.

If you are currently overweight, out of shape, and have attempted a plan that failed, then realize you were treating your situation with the wrong prescription. You either didn't formulate a prescription, or the one you had wasn't effective. Your prescription, or what you do during the time you allocate to exercise, is an essential element to your plan's success.

Let's begin by creating a new prescription for you. The principal difference between your former prescription and your new one is that from this point forth, you will devote 25 percent of your workout time to cardiovascular exercise and 75 percent to strength and resistance training. I know that this is contrary to most exercise programs, which stress heavily, if not exclusively, cardiovascular exercise. But let's face it, the vast majority of these programs aren't getting the job done.

Is cardiovascular exercise beneficial to your body? Of course. Your heart is the single most important muscle of the body, and doing cardiovascular exercise will help to preserve that muscle. But is cardiovascular exercise an efficient way to preserve lean muscle tissue? *No.* One study reported that even men who run regularly still lost nearly five pounds of muscle in their upper body over the course of ten years. In order to lose weight, we must preserve muscle throughout the entire body, both upper and lower, and only strength and resistance training will accomplish that. The only exception to this would be elite athletes who perform cardiovascular exercise at an incredible frequency, duration, and intensity. Do you ice skate as frequently and with the intensity of Olympic gold medalist Dan Jansen, or do you bicycle with the frequency and intensity of Tour de France winner Lance Armstrong?

CARDIOVASCULAR EXERCISE ALONE IS NOT THE ANSWER

Like most individuals, when you initiated an exercise program, you took up walking, bought a treadmill, or maybe you even purchased one of the machines hyped on late-night infomercials. It seemed like the easiest solution. We all know how to walk, and the idea of approaching a strength and resistance program is daunting for most people. So you started your program by walking. Did you stick with this walking program? If you purchased another piece of cardiovascular equipment, did you use your Health Rider, stair stepper, bike, cross-country machine, or rower? Did you see lasting results? Did you lose weight? No.

In 1987 there were 4.4 million treadmill users. Guess what the number was in 1998? A whopping 37.1 million. Americans continue their love affair with treadmills, so why are we getting fatter and fatter every year?

Let's consider the issue of internal versus external forces. Cardiovascular exercise is an *external* force that periodically boosts your metabolism for a limited period of time and enables you to burn additional calories. Strength and resistance training *internally* boosts your metabolism and enables you to burn additional calories *twenty-four hours* a day. Why not pick a stimulus that works internally and around the clock rather than something that works externally and only for brief periods of time?

Here is another way to appreciate the benefits of strength and resistance training. As we age, especially by our twenties and thirties, we begin to lose muscle. Think of your strength and resistance program as a way to regain what you once had, and rebuild a strong *internal* metabolic system.

Why, then, devote even 25 percent of your exercise prescription to cardiovascular exercise? Why not devote all of it to strength and resistance training? Cardiovascular exercise does challenge the most important muscle of the body—the heart. When you go for a walk, or get on a treadmill, bike, stair machine, or elliptical trainer, the large muscles of the lower body, predominately the front of the legs (quadriceps), back of the legs (hamstrings), and buttocks (gluteus maximus), require oxygen to perform the activity. Oxygen is transported to the muscles by the blood, and the blood is pumped by the heart. So when you begin to exercise, your heart rate elevates to supply the increased amount of oxygen to the working muscles. Two variables play a role in how much elevation occurs within the heart: your fitness level and the intensity of the exercise.

STRENGTH AND RESISTANCE TRAINING BOOSTS YOUR METABOLISM

As a beginner, the heart is not used to the activity you are performing, and subsequently will be surprised by the need to supply oxygen to the working muscles. Say you climb a flight of stairs and find yourself at the top gasping for breath. What happened? Well, the heart began pumping and could not get the necessary amount of oxygen to the working muscles, so you start to gasp for breath in an attempt to take in more oxygen. Your circulatory system is not used to transporting blood/oxygen in this manner, and the heart's stroke volume, or the amount of blood pumped each beat, is low. With time and consistent training, these factors will improve and you will experience the *training effect*—basically, you will be more in shape. In other words, improved cardiovascularity translates to a more efficient blood/oxygen transportation system. That is why my program devotes 25 percent of your exercise time to preserving the most important muscle in the body, the heart. But that's all you need. Recall my remarks in Chapter 2, Fallacy 6, "I'm fat but fit." True, through cardiovascular exercise an overweight individual can perform many activities that require a strong heart and efficient cardiovascular functioning. But being in better cardiovascular shape does not necessarily translate into being in the weight-loss business. You must strength-and-resistance train in order to be in the weight-loss business.

The American Medical Association states that twenty minutes of cardiovascular exercise three times a week can yield signifi-

The Business Plan for the Body

cant benefits and strengthen the heart muscle. But more than that is truly unnecessary if your goal is permanent weight reduction. Keep that goal in your head: permanent weight reduction. Now, if your mission statement is, "I want to improve my ability to walk on a treadmill," then walk on a treadmill. If your mission statement is, "I want to improve my ability to ride a bicycle," then ride a bike. Just realize, you are not in the weight-loss business, you are in the treadmill-walking or bicycle-riding business. What business do you wish to be in?

One additional reason to perform cardiovascular exercise is due to the aging process. As we age, our aerobic capacity begins to diminish. Some studies have shown that by the age of ninety, most people who don't exercise would lose 50 percent of their aerobic capacity. By including cardiovascular exercise, you can minimize that reduction in capacity to about 5 percent. Fifty percent diminishment or 5 percent. That is within your power.

YOUR HEART ONLY NEEDS TWENTY MINUTES OF CARDIO THREE TIMES A WEEK

When you do cardiovascular exercise, your body burns calories at an accelerated rate. The following chart gives an indication of approximately how many calories are burned through various exercises.

APPROXIMATE CALORIES BURNED DURING 30 MINUTES OF PHYSICAL ACTIVITY

TYPE OF ACTIVITY	130-POUND ADULT	175-POUND ADULT
Walking	130	180
Cycling	180	240
Swimming	210	300
Jogging	300	400
In-line Skating	210	280
Aerobic Dance	180	240
Singles Tennis	180	270
Frisbee	180	240
Skiing	240	330
Weight Lifting	210	240

Please keep in mind that these are approximations, as an individual's lean muscle tissue, age, weight, fitness level, genetic predisposition, and numerous other factors need to be taken into consideration in order to get the exact number of calories burned. Note the calories burned through weight lifting. It burns almost as many calories as other activities, but only weight lifting comes with the added twenty-four-hour-a-day metabolic boost; you burn additional calories around the clock. Consider that again. You can perform many physical activities, but only weight training burns additional calories while you are performing the activity *and* burns additional calories twenty-four hours a day, due to the increase in lean muscle tissue that it creates!

I am positive you are thinking, "What about the number of calories the treadmill tells me I burned each time I exercise?" That number is only an average. Look at the facts. Get on a treadmill and punch in 175 pounds. Are you a 175-pound, fifty-five-year-old, out-of-shape woman? A 175-pound, ten-year-old obese child? Or a 175-pound, thirty-nine-year-old man in good shape? Each will burn a different number of calories; how much will depend mostly upon the elevation of each person's heart rate, age, genetic predisposition, lean muscle tissue, etc. The manufacturer of the equipment is simply trying to provide a gauge, which unfortunately is usually incorrect. People like to see this gauge and proudly proclaim, "I burned x number of calories on the treadmill," when that is rarely the case. This is one instance where one size does not fit all. And again, you aren't building lean muscle tissue.

Regardless of the calories the machine states you have expended, most individuals exercise, then negate all the calories burned with one bagel, one double latte, one scone, or way too many ounces of frozen yogurt. You must balance your energy in with your energy out. Believing a cardiovascular machine that tells you that you burned 650 calories, then going out and eating all the wrong foods in the wrong quantities, will only lead to further weight gain, not weight loss.

Research by Dr. Michelle Olson of Auburn University suggests that "the overwhelming majority of the time, exercise machines tend to overestimate calories by as much as 20 to 30 percent." So please don't believe the machines.

Let's go back to my anecdote at the beginning of this chapter, and my urging you to visit the cardio room and the strength and resistance room of a health club. Quickly run back into the cardio room and make yet another observation. How many people are "hanging" onto their machine—usually the treadmill,

StairMaster, and elliptical trainer? The majority are. According to Steve Farrell of the Cooper Institute for Aerobics Research in Dallas, Texas, "Leaning on the handrails of a stair climber or keeping a 'death grip' on the treadmill railing will greatly decrease your caloric expenditure. The machine is assuming that your legs are carrying your entire body weight. By supporting yourself, you are probably burning 20 to 30 percent *fewer* calories than the machine indicates." In addition to reduced caloric burning, you are also impairing your posture by not utilizing your abdominals and lower back for support, and probably hurting your back, shoulders, and neck. So, no hanging on to the equipment, please. If you have to hold on, you are working at too high an intensity level and deluding yourself into believing that you're burning more calories by jacking the intensity level up.

It is imperative to know your heart rate when you exercise. You can take a manual heart rate at your wrist or neck, but one of the best exercise equipment investments you can make is in a heart rate monitor, which is a simple, easy-to-use device. By placing a strap around your chest that transmits to a watch on your wrist, you know at all times exactly how your heart is responding to exercise. If you have recently been in an exercise equipment store, you may have noticed that the majority of new cardiovascular equipment is manufactured with a built-in heart rate monitor. All you have to do is wear the chest strap, which transmits directly to the machine. Some of these machines can even be programmed so you tell the computer at what heart rate you desire to exercise, and the machine will go faster or slower, or increase or decrease the incline.

KNOW YOUR HEART RATE

If you do not have a heart rate monitor, then take a fifteen-second manual pulse at your wrist or neck and multiply that number by four to get your sixty-second heart rate. Start counting from zero instead of one. Place your index finger at your wrist and begin your fifteen-second count with 0, 1, 2, . . . Multiply that number by four, and there you have it. Take this manual reading every seven to ten minutes to obtain a gauge of how your heart rate is responding to the exercise. This is invaluable information, and so necessary to establishing a starting point and applying *progression*. Remember that word, *progression*. In Chapter 9 we will discuss it in great detail.

The following equation is used to determine maximum heart rate:

$$220 \text{ Minus Your Age} = \text{Maximum Heart Rate}$$

One should never strive to exercise at maximum heart rate, but rather, use it to obtain a target heart rate. Once you have determined your maximum heart rate, you then take a percentage of it. For those of you who are beginners, you may shoot for a target heart rate between 60 and 70 percent of your maximum heart rate; intermediate exercisers, 70 to 80 percent of your maximum heart rate; and advanced exercisers may shoot for an intensity up to 85 percent of your maximum heart rate. If I use myself as an example, at forty years old, my equation would be:

220 – 40 (my age) = 180 (my maximum heart rate)

60% times 180 (maximum heart rate) = 108

70% times 180 (maximum heart rate) = 126

80% times 180 (maximum heart rate) = 144

85% times 180 (maximum heart rate) = 153

This information then enables me to determine at what intensity level I wish to work. This equation is only an approximation. Most of us should just listen to our bodies when exercising and adjust the intensity level accordingly. I simply included the equation to give you direction.

In addition to the intensity of the exercise, two other variables determine how many calories one burns through cardiovascular exercise. The first is *duration,* how long you keep your heart rate elevated; and the second is *frequency,* how many times a week you do cardiovascular exercise.

Briefly let me touch upon the subject of exercise intensity and burning fat. The entire issue of burning fat is vastly misunderstood. There are two sources of fuel the body uses to exercise: fat and carbohydrate. The media have led us to believe that the lower the intensity, say 60 percent of your maximum heart rate, the greater percentage of fuel for the exercise will come from fat; the higher the intensity, the greater the percentage will come from carbohydrate. This is true. What is also true is that

The Business Plan for the Body

the higher the intensity of the exercise, the more calories burned. I want you to think *burn calories* and stop worrying about the fuel source. Research has shown that if you burn fat during exercise, you will burn carbohydrate during the rest of the day, and vice versa. It simply does not matter what fuel source is used. "The idea that you can't lose fat unless you burn fat while you exercise has absolutely no scientific support," says Jeffrey Rupp, Ph.D., Georgia State University. Please, just think "calories expended." Remember, *creating a caloric deficit is the key to weight loss.*

We know that cardiovascular exercise is important to the preservation of the heart muscle and our aerobic capacity, and have established that cardiovascular exercise has a place in your prescription, but as I said, that place should equal 25 percent of your allotted exercise time. You know you have tried a heavy cardiovascular exercise prescription in the past. It didn't work. Go back to my opening observation. Put this book down, go to the nearest health club or fitness facility, walk into the cardiovascular room, then into the strength and resistance room, and draw your own conclusion. As you draw that conclusion, consider the following.

Most respondents to a national survey say they exercise regularly, but few do anything more vigorous than walking. We know that as Americans, we have ballooned in size, so, is the walking and other cardiovascular activity keeping us lean? Obviously not.

But it is necessary to allocate 25 percent of your exercise time to cardiovascular exercise.

EXAMPLES OF CARDIOVASCULAR ACTIVITIES
IN YOUR HOME OR OUTDOORS

Walking, either in place or outside; jogging or running; climbing stairs in your home, apartment building, or up and down a single step; bike riding, swimming, dancing, or low-impact aerobics to music or a videotape. All can successfully elevate your heart rate, depending on the intensity.

EXAMPLES OF CARDIOVASCULAR EXERCISE
IN A GYM OR EXERCISE FACILITY

Treadmill, bike, stair stepper, elliptical trainer, rowing machine, ergometer, swimming, or VersaClimber. Once again, all can successfully elevate your heart rate depending on the intensity.

So, we are in agreement. Seventy-five percent of your allotted exercise time should be devoted to strength and resistance training. Besides building lean muscle tissue, the additional benefits of strength and resistance training are as follows:

ADDITIONAL BENEFITS OF STRENGTH AND RESISTANCE TRAINING

Burn additional calories. As you saw from the chart of calories burned for thirty minutes of exercise, weight lifting burned more calories than cycling. And remember, when you weight-train, you get the benefit of increased caloric burning similar to cardiovascular exercise, plus a twenty-four-hour-a-day postmetabolic boost through the creation of lean muscle tissue. How could you justify doing any other form of exercise?

Increase strength throughout the entire body. This is great for everyday activities such as carrying groceries, children, briefcases, etc. Many formerly stressful situations, such as carrying luggage to your car or placing it in an overhead compartment on an airplane, become vastly easier and less taxing.

Decrease chance of injury, as your muscles become stronger and more flexible. So often, we hear about bad shoulders from golf or tennis, stiff necks or muscle atrophy. As you become stronger and more flexible, you will feel much better and forestall many of the common problems associated with muscle atrophy, imbalance, and aging.

Increase joint stability and flexibility, which diminishes the effect of arthritis. One hundred twenty-five forms of arthritis affect nearly fifty million Americans. Rheumatoid arthritis, one of the most severe forms, affects 1 percent of the population. We all experience some arthritis as we age. Strength and resistance training increases strength in the tendons, ligaments, and muscles surrounding our joints, which lessens the pain and improves the functioning of those joints. A study at Boston University also showed that a "weight loss of eleven

BECOME STRONGER AND MORE FLEXIBLE

pounds or more lowered the risk for developing osteoarthritis in the knee by as much as 50 percent." In addition, studies have indicated that a person with arthritis who exercises can wind up in better shape than a sedentary individual with normal joints.

Prevent lower back problems and strengthen your "core." Strength and resistance training can dramatically strengthen your lower back, abdominals, and muscles throughout your body and improve the balance in your "core," or the foundation of your body. A study, described in *Consumer Reports on Health,* of over six hundred individuals—who had already tried an average of six treatment methods for their chronic back pain—found that 70 percent of those in a back-strengthening program experienced substantial relief.

Improved bone mineral density and reduced risk of osteoporosis, joint replacements, and other related disorders. Presently, ten million Americans, 80 percent of them women, suffer from osteoporosis, or thinning of the bones. In addition, another eighteen million have low bone mass, commonly referred to as osteopenia, a precursor to osteoporosis. The National Osteoporosis Foundation predicts that number will soar to forty-one million over the next fifteen years due to the aging of baby boomers. Regular strength and resistance training is not an option, it is a necessity, as repeated stress on the bones by strength and resistance training *improves* density and *does not* weaken them. According to Dr. Joseph Lane, head of the Osteoporosis Prevention Center at the Hospital for Special Surgery in New York City, "I've seen women in their eighties increase their bone mass up to 10 percent a year with a simple weight-lifting regimen."

Decreased total serum cholesterol, and especially the LDL or "bad" cholesterol. Over 100 million Americans now have high cholesterol. A recent study showed that regular strength and resistance training reduced total cholesterol by 10 percent and the LDL, or bad cholesterol, by 14 percent.

Improved glucose metabolism, or blood sugar functioning, which diminishes the risk of Type II diabetes. Sixteen million Americans suffer from diabetes, and close to 95 percent of those sixteen million have Type II, or adult onset, diabetes. To make matters worse, of the sixteen million diabetics, only one-half are aware of their condition. Diabetes ranks as the fourth leading cause of death in the United States. In addition, the incidence of Type II diabetes in children is increasing at an astonishing rate as a result of obesity and inactivity. Increased muscle mass improves the body's ability to use insulin more efficiently in processing sugar out of the blood and moving it through tissue where it is expended as energy. The less insulin that is required to perform this function, the more plentiful the insulin supply will be throughout life.

Reduce the risk of colon cancer. Muscle building brings improved intestinal transit time. Tests have shown that weight training can halve gastrointestinal transit time. The faster waste passes through the colon, the less probability that carcinogens will remain in your system and attach to the intestinal wall.

Reduces high blood pressure. A recent study reported by the American Heart Association's journal, *Hypertensions,* showed that strength training does indeed take pressure off the circulatory system. "This was controversial for years," says the study's lead author, George Kelley, associate professor of exercise science at Northern Illinois University. "People thought weight training could actually increase blood pressure. Not so." After three months of strength training, systolic blood pressure, or force generated against artery walls during contraction, decreased by 2 percent, and diastolic pressure, the force generated against artery walls during relaxation, dropped 4 percent. While these benefits may seem modest, they significantly reduce the risk of stroke and heart disease.

Improved posture and overall appearance. Properly executed strength and resistance training can significantly improve your posture. Observe yourself in the mirror and assess your posture. You have to love the visual changes that occur when you throw your shoulders back and tuck your abdominals. Strength and resistance training can also give your body a more symmetrical appearance.

Less risk of falls for the elderly. We have established that strength and resistance exercise can increase your bone density and muscular strength. One of the primary reasons the elderly are injured is because of falls. By improving balance, strength, and flexibility, many of these falls can be prevented or the result of a fall can be minimized. Also, keep in mind, we always hear about elderly men and women who fall and break their hip. Frequently, the opposite is true. The hip actually breaks first, because of diminished bone density, and then the individual falls. In some bone density scans, a hip can be as thin as a golf tee. For the senior population, strength and resistance training is not an option. It is a ticket to an independent, injury-free life. The same applies to the younger population. They, too, can minimize the risk of falls, avoid injury, and enhance their sense of balance.

Increased energy. According to Miriam E. Nelson, author of *Strong Women Stay Thin,* in addition to all the benefits of strength and resistance training previously discussed, participants who strength-trained for one year were energized. "They became 27 percent more active and their bodies were fifteen to twenty years more youthful." Mind you, this was after only one year of strength training.

If you still are convinced that a strength and resistance training program is not for you, allow me to address some of the common misconceptions that may have erroneously led you to that position.

QUESTIONS AND COMMON MISCONCEPTIONS REGARDING STRENGTH AND RESISTANCE TRAINING

Won't I hurt myself doing strength and resistance training? No. On the contrary, if you follow the instructions in *The Business Plan for the Body,* review the enclosed illustrations, concentrate and listen to your body, you will be safely performing the exercises, and actually improve what is called the "structural integrity" of the body. The "structural integrity" of the body pertains to posture, balance, and alignment. Frequently, injury occurs within the body because of muscular imbalance, whether it be weak abdominals, which can lead to lower back problems, overdeveloped quadriceps (front of the leg), or underdeveloped hamstrings (back of the leg), which frequently lead to knee problems, in addition to other imbalances. Even the American College of Sports Medicine says low back pain is generally attributed to abdominal muscle weakness and poor flexibility in the low back–hamstring region. Properly prescribed resistance training can strengthen both the abdominal and lumbar extensors, which support and protect the spine. Strength training is the only activity that improves imbalance. Research at Colorado State University has shown that the benefits of strength training exercise far outweighs the risks of injury if done correctly. Or as you have heard so many times. "If you don't use it, you lose it."

Won't I bulk up? Absolutely not. The muscle-building potential of men is enhanced by the presence of testosterone, but even with testosterone, it is very difficult to build so much muscle that an individual actually becomes bulky. Women, without the benefit of similar testosterone levels, clearly have very little chance of ever bulking up. The problem is all the bodybuilder magazines or fitness programs that show or depict individuals with a tremendous amount of muscular development, which they probably acquired predominantly with the assistance of illegal supplements and an extreme eating and exercise regime. That does not apply to you or me.

I only want to "tone" my muscles, not build them up. What is the right program for me? Let me be perfectly clear. There is no such thing as "toning" a muscle. I believe what most people are interested in when they say they want to "tone" a muscle is to see a long, lean, visible muscle with very little body fat camouflaging that muscle; think, ballet dancers. Let's use the arm muscle as an example, because women over and over ask my staff or me to prescribe exercises to firm up their upper arms. We repeatedly explain that we must build the arm muscles in conjunction with building lean muscle tissue throughout the body in order to increase basal metabolic rate, burn additional calories twenty-four hours a day, and therefore reduce body fat content. That is the only way to achieve the results they desire. Only two variables dictate the appearance of the front muscle of the arm, the bicep, and the back muscle of the arm muscle, the tricep. The first variable is the size of the muscle. We know that after the age of twenty the average person loses seven-tenths of a pound of muscle a year. We know that

The Business Plan for the Body

only through strength and resistance training can you increase the size, or presence, of that muscle and reverse that trend. Therefore, to get the long, lean visual in the arm, you need to do strength and resistance training to build or rebuild the muscle. Variable two is the percentage of body fat. If you are overweight, or possess too much fat on your arm, you will not be able to see the muscle because it is covered by body fat.

Think about Michelangelo's David at the Accademia in Florence, Italy. Nearly everyone has seen at least a copy, if not the original, of this incredible sculpture of a young man with sharp muscular definition. I often say to my clients who are familiar with the sculpture, "What if you put fifteen pounds of body fat over David's muscles? The muscles would still be there, but we wouldn't be able to see them." So, if you want to be "toned," you must strength- and resistance-train to build the muscle *and* reduce your body fat content through strength and resistance training and the proper diet. This will make the muscle you have developed more apparent and will produce the so-called toning effect.

A brief note for those of you who are at an ideal weight and do not see any muscular development on your body. It is possible to be at an acceptable weight, or even underweight (which applies to many anorexic and bulimic individuals), and not be muscularly defined. Most likely this has occurred because you have not embraced a progressive, consistent, strength and resistance program. You may be doing cardiovascular exercise and wondering why your muscles don't show. I personally see many runners up and down Lake Shore Drive in Chicago, men and women, who clearly are in good cardiovascular condition with low body weight, but who definitely possess a high percentage of body fat, which is noticeable in their abs, arms, hips, gluts, and thighs. They are neglecting the most important element of exercise. Only through strength and resistance training will you ever develop muscle, boost your metabolism twenty-four hours a day, burn body fat, and have the opportunity to see the results of your effort.

Isn't it true that to build muscle I have to lift heavy weight for fewer repetitions, and if I only want to build endurance, or "tone" my muscles, I should do less weight and more repetitions? Absolutely not. This is a question I am frequently asked when people hear I am in the fitness industry. Fact: To stimulate a muscle through strength and resistance training, you must "overload" that muscle. What is "overload"? There are basically three phases your muscle experiences as you perform a set of repetitions of a particular exercise. Phase one, "working repetitions," constitutes about 75 percent of the portion of each set. A set traditionally consists of twelve to fifteen repetitions of the same exercise. With relative ease, you are able to perform a certain number of repetitions of the movement in good form. Phase two, approximately the next 20 percent, begins when you start to experience some discomfort, or slight burn, in the muscle, and the exercise becomes harder to execute. Your muscle is going into "fatigue." You may also be tempted to cheat, or enlist other muscles into helping you perform the movement. This is why your form becomes so important. Phase three, you hit "failure," or momentary muscular inability to perform the activity.

At this point you are finished with your set. The muscle does not know if you achieved failure with heavy weight and few repetitions, or less weight and more repetitions. All the muscle knows is that in thirty to ninety seconds it will go through all three phases, working repetitions, fatigue, and ultimately experience failure. Once the muscle hits failure, the exercise is over, but the process of building muscle is just beginning.

MUSCLE BUILDING OCCURS AFTER EXERCISE

This building process occurs *after* the exercise. Yes, *after* the exercise. During the set, you are challenging the muscle and forcing it to perform beyond its current capabilities. As you go through the three exercise phases, you conclude with failure, or the muscle's temporary inability to continue the movement. This sets the muscle-building process in motion. When you failed to perform the final repetitions, you stressed the muscle and created tiny tears in the muscle tissue. Simultaneously, a signal is sent to the brain saying, "I need some help down here. I want to be able to lift that weight with greater ease the next time I am asked to perform this activity. So help me grow." This is followed by the repair phase. The muscle begins the repair process, which leads to growth. Over the next twenty-four to forty-eight hours, the tiny tears will repair and, since the brain is telling the body that it wants to perform the exercise with greater efficiency the next time it's called upon, the muscle will repair with *additional* muscle tissue in order to be stronger. Remember this correlation. More muscle, more strength; more strength, more muscle. They always go hand in hand. That is the process your body experiences when you participate in a strength and resistance program. You build strength, you build muscle. You overload a muscle, create tiny tears in the muscle tissue, and stimulate the muscle to repair. The repair occurs at *rest*. Then, as we will explore in Chapter 9, you must progress the muscular overload to continue to achieve growth.

For those of you put off by the concept of creating tiny tears in the muscle, don't be. This is the process your body goes through to build muscle. It is a positive phenomenon, not a negative.

Now, regarding our previous discussion, the muscle does not know if it was stressed with a low-rep, high-weight program to build muscle, or a high-rep, low-weight program to "tone" the muscle. Do you see how this is impossible? All the muscle knows is that it has been challenged. Since the human body is very intelligent, the body wants to meet the challenge. The muscle responds to stimuli. You are stimulating the muscle by executing a progressive, consistent plan, placing stress on the muscle for thirty to ninety seconds. High reps, low reps; high weight, low weight; who cares? Your body doesn't. All it cares about is the three phases, performed safely, in good form, with relaxed breathing. The goal here is to build muscle. Period.

Won't I lose flexibility if I lift weights? No. Proper strength and resistance training can actually improve flexibility and muscular balance. This concept is called *reciprocal inhibition*. In lay terms, it means that when you contract, for example, the bicep muscle in the front of the arm, the tricep muscle at the back of the arm has to relax, elongate, and stretch out. Basically, when you contract one muscle, you stretch the opposing one. This clearly will improve flexibility over time. Another variable with regard to flexibility is balance. As you will see when we develop the exercise plan, our program is about muscular balance that promotes flexibility.

Don't I need to buy a lot of expensive exercise equipment? No, a minimal amount of equipment and expenditure is required to begin a comprehensive program. Later in this chapter I will elaborate on equipment specifics.

Won't this type of program take forever to produce results? No. As muscles are challenged, they must adapt, and that does not take much time. According to Tufts University, individuals in their nineties can triple their strength and increase lean muscle tissue 10 percent after just eight weeks of strength training three times a week. And remember, with an increase in strength, you will have a corresponding increase in lean muscle tissue. Strength training for three months can increase the BMR rate by 7 percent. Briefly, this is but yet another reason to embrace strength and resistance training. You will definitely see results in a minimal amount of time. It is quite exciting to step out of the shower, glimpse your body, which you may have been reluctant to do in the past, and like what you see: good posture, improved muscular development, your body composition changing. This will motivate you to continue. When you only do cardiovascular exercise, your only hope is to reduce your size, not change your shape. Look at your body right now. Would you be happy with the same shape just a little smaller? I hope your answer is no. You want to be smaller with the best composition your body will allow. Only strength and resistance training will sculpt one's body, improve posture and bone mass, which translates into maintaining one's height.

NOTICEABLE RESULTS IN MINIMAL TIME

Won't this require a lot of my time? No. Most people can achieve significant benefits with three sessions a week, which is the optimal amount of time to devote to strength and resistance training. But if all your schedule will allow is twice a week, then you could derive 75 percent of the benefits of training three times a week. Over the years, I have personally worked with individuals who initially began their exercise program twice a week. When the client increased to three or more sessions a week, the results achieved were quite dramatic. So plan on a minimum of two sessions a week, but do plan in the future to increase that allocation. Given the fact that a week consists of 168 hours, two hours isn't much!

Don't I have to join an expensive health club? No. The exercise plan I recommend can be done in the convenience of your home or office and can easily be taken on the road. Remember this expression: "It's not the equipment, it is the application." I have seen people with $100,000 exercise rooms in their homes who look and feel terrible. I have also seen people with some free weights and exercise tubing, a couple of hundred dollars or

The Business Plan for the Body

less of equipment, look terrific. Also, current research reveals that individuals working out in their homes tend to be much more consistent with their programs than those who must travel to an exercise facility.

I'm confused. One person tells me that free weights are best for building muscle and another tells me it's machines. Who is correct? Actually, neither. As I just said, it is not the equipment, it's the application of the equipment. Here is a brief analysis of free weights versus machines. Using a chest press exercise as an illustration, with free weights, you lie on a bench, place a dumbbell in each hand, and slowly press up. Your body has to work to both control the weight, preventing it from going sideways, and press the weight up and down. In using a chest press machine, you lie down or sit in the machine and are only required to press the weight up and down or forward and back. You do not have to stabilize the weight because the machine does it for you. Which exercise is better? That is not easily answered. So many other variables come into play, such as form, speed, resistance level, and the size of the equipment versus the size of the individual. All variables being constant, the free weight will force the muscle to work a little harder because it has to control the weight.

The benefit of machines? For beginners, it is easier to control the weight and may be a "safer" option if you fit correctly into the machine. And for some exercises, you need a machine since the free weights or tubing cannot duplicate the motion. The benefit of free weights and tubing? First, you control the range of motion, not the machine. Second, you have to control the weight or tube, which leads to increased muscle fiber recruitment. So what is the answer? Neither. It is how the exercise is performed. We are starting with light resistance, correct form and posture. At this point it doesn't matter whether it is with machines or free weights.

Do I have to give up my walks on the beach or weekend bike rides since you urge me not to do so much cardiovascular exercise? No. If you enjoy playing tennis, walking, biking, swimming, or any other similar activity, go ahead and do them. Just realize, I still expect you to perform a minimum of two and ideally three or four strength and resistance training sessions each week. If these activities you enjoy are in addition to the strength and resistance training, fine. If they are in lieu of the strength and resistance training, then you are not following the recommended *Business Plan for the Body* guidelines to successful weight loss.

Isn't this type of strength and resistance program complicated? No. As you will see in the next section, my strength and resistance program is very easy to execute.

THE THREE ESSENTIAL COMPONENTS TO A STRENGTH AND RESISTANCE PROGRAM

COMPONENT ONE—SPECIFICITY

You want to be very specific about the muscle you are isolating. I touched upon this concept in our discussion of high reps, low reps, high weight versus light weight. As you are performing a strength and resistance exercise, your muscle proceeds from working repetitions, into fatigue, and ultimately failure. As you are tiring, other muscles will attempt to step in to assist the working muscle with the movement. You don't want to allow that, as it will take the stress off the muscle you are trying to isolate and stimulate. Be conscious of your form. Concentrate on the muscle you are working. Studies have proven that the more you think about the muscle contracting and releasing, the more you will stimulate and recruit the muscle fiber. An old weight lifter expression is, "Link the mind to the muscle." I totally agree. Specificity. Remember that word.

COMPONENT TWO—OVERLOAD

You must overload a muscle to force it to grow. Either through weight, repetitions, sets, speed (the slower the speed of the movement, the greater the resistance on the muscle), or stability—performing an exercise on an unstable surface, such as a ball or board, is more difficult; a muscle must be overloaded in order to grow. Confusion facilitates change. Overloading a muscle confuses it and stimulates it to grow. A muscle is overloaded as it goes from fatigue to failure. If you can perform an exercise with ease, you are not overloading the muscle. The exercise has hit a plateau. To create a new overload, the program must embrace component three, progression.

COMPONENT THREE—PROGRESSION

Chapter 9 is entirely devoted to the concept of progression. You must "progress" both a cardiovascular and a strength and resistance program in order to continually achieve additional results. Since we know that the body, through the aging process, tends to lose muscle and diminish in aerobic capacity, we must constantly challenge and progress the program so we do not allow that to occur.

Now, let's move forward and outline the specifics of your new exercise plan.

THE STRATEGIC EXERCISE PLAN

1. SCHEDULING

For the first three months, you agree to spend a minimum of two, preferably three separate hours a week exercising. Get out your scheduling book and make the appointments with yourself, or if you are going to use a fitness trainer or exercise partner, then arrange the sessions now. I want you to make your exercise sessions a priority. If you wait to fit exercise in after everything else, you and I know it will not happen. You are in the weight-loss business. The only way to successfully remain viable in the weight-loss business is to exercise.

Every successful client I or my firm has ever worked with has one common denominator: all religiously scheduled and attended sessions. Let me give you an example: Say you are a regular Monday, Wednesday, Friday client of my firm. You are going away for a long weekend. The successful weight-loss client calls my office and leaves the following message. "I am going out of town for a long weekend so I have to miss my Friday session this week and the Monday after. Could you please schedule me for Thursday of this week and Tuesday of the following? I want to make sure to get my three sessions in." That's a recipe for success. I know this client is committed to the weight-loss business and will see results.

Now, here's the unsuccessful client. "I have to be out of town on Friday and Monday so cancel those two sessions. You know, I am going to be so busy before going away, I had better also cancel the Wednesday before and the Wednesday after. Come to think of it, take me off the schedule book for the next two weeks and I will call you when I want to resume my training."

Wrong, wrong, wrong. You are never going to successfully be in the weight-loss business if you do not make exercise a priority and carve out the necessary time to accomplish your goals. How many businesses do you

MAKE EXERCISE A PRIORITY

know that just close shop for two weeks and expect their clients, customers, vendors, and employees to understand? Not many I know of. So schedule, and do it before you load up your time with work, family, friends, and other interests. You must maintain focus.

There is a couple in my condominium building with two seven-year-old twin boys. Almost every morning, the husband comes down to the building exercise room before his wife, he either swims or lifts weights, then goes upstairs. Minutes later his wife arrives for her workout. It is a perfect setup. She starts the kids off in the morning, breakfast, getting dressed, etc., while her husband is exercising. Then the moment he returns, she is dressed and ready to go down for her exercise session, and he finishes with the kids and gets himself ready for work. Both husband and wife consistently exercise. Now these workouts may only be thirty or forty minutes during the week. Doing a full hour is perhaps not realistic. However, on the weekends I see them both getting more exercise time in to make sure that they stay in shape. As I frequently talk with them, each makes the point of saying, "We use this exercise for both the physical and mental benefits. Two seven-year-olds require energy and patience. We both feel the regular exercise really helps."

You, too, can make the time to exercise. Stop and think for a moment. If necessary, get out your daily planner, Palm Pilot, whatever you use to keep your schedule. First, decide to make exercise a priority. As I have said over and over, if you don't embrace exercise in your plan, you are not serious about going into the weight-loss business. Possibly, exercise may fit in your current schedule without many adjustments. If not, then you *must* decide what you are going to delete, or rearrange, in order to meet this crucial component of the weight-loss business, exercise. I am positive you *can* come up with a schedule that makes exercise a reality in your life.

Ideally, you will schedule exercise every other day. If your schedule does not permit this protocol, then you can modify the

The Business Plan for the Body

program if you must do back-to-back sessions. The reason for every-other-day exercise relates to rest. As mentioned earlier, when we perform strength and resistance training, we are not actually building lean muscle tissue, the building occurs during rest. Remember, what happens is that during strength and resistance training, you are creating tiny tears in the muscle tissue as force, or resistance, is applied against the muscle. That's the overload I previously mentioned. After this stress has occurred, the muscle, through various neurological and physiological responses, will grow larger and subsequently stronger. For most big muscle groups, such as the back, chest, and legs, approximately forty-eight hours is the optimal time for rest. For smaller muscles, including the abdominals, twenty-four hours is enough. You can do cardiovascular exercise every day, since the stress to the muscles is minimal though even daily cardiovascular exercise will not put you in the weight-loss business.

Everyone should always take one complete day off a week from all exercise to allow the body to completely repair. Since we are starting our program with full body workouts, then every-other-day exercise is ideal. However, if it is necessary for you to exercise on back-to-back days, then you will modify your prescription, which I will discuss in Chapter 9. Don't be concerned if you have to exercise on back-to-back days. Many of our successful clients, who travel extensively for business during the week, always schedule both Saturday and Sunday and effectively get the job done.

2. ALLOCATION

Remember, plan to allocate 25 percent of your time to cardiovascular exercise and 75 percent of the time to strength and resistance training. If you plan to exercise for an hour, that translates to approximately fifteen minutes of cardiovascular each session followed by forty-five minutes of strength and resistance training. If you plan to exercise more or less, adjust the time accordingly. Keep in mind, walking, running, cycling, or stair stepping is not the only way to keep your heart rate elevated. During weight training, your heart will be elevated, but probably not to the extent it was during your cardiovascular exercise. Don't forget, muscles require oxygen in order to perform activity, so strength training will keep your heart rate elevated as well.

Within your 75 percent strength and resistance allocation, plan to spend two-thirds of your time on exercises for the back of the body and one-third on exercises for the front of the body. Let me repeat: Two-thirds of your strength and resistance training should be targeted to the back of the body, not the front of your body. More on this subject later, when we design your exercise program in detail.

3. ASSESS YOUR WEAKNESSES OR INJURIES

In the past, if you have experienced a joint or muscular problem, such as a bad knee or back, plan on doing some rehabilitation of those areas. Start by rereading the exercises a physical therapist probably gave you that you neglected to perform. If you didn't consult a doctor or physical therapist for the problem, then make an appointment to do so now. Remember, don't start a program with an injury or imbalance that goes unattended or undiagnosed. You are beginning a lifelong exercise plan, so you want to start out strong.

Let me elaborate on this issue. I always use the following analogy with my clients: Say you are making a business decision to expand your corporate headquarters, redesign your warehouse, or renovate your restaurant. The first step is to have an architect or engineer assess the integrity of the space, such as the foundation, wiring, plumbing, etc. You would never just rip out walls and add rooms unless you knew the structure could internally withstand the changes. Think of your body as being under renovation. It is, after all, your "corporate headquarters." Why begin a program with structural problems left unaddressed or unattended? If you do neglect these "weak links" in your body, then I guarantee the injury will get worse and ultimately force you to break down and cease exercising. This is not the goal. The goal is to add exercise for the rest of your life, so don't miss this crucial step. If you are injured or feel specific pain, call your doctor. Make the appointment. Follow up with therapy or whatever instructions you receive. Improve the "structural integrity" of your body.

4. RECORDING

Invest in a notebook to record your exercise progress. This could easily be the same notebook in which you record your food diary and, as you will learn in subsequent chapters, your

The Business Plan for the Body

weekly weight. Remember, one of the most essential elements to the plan is progression. Progression requires documentation. If you don't record the data, how will you know how to appropriately take your plan to the next level? Would you invest in a stock or business that supplied absolutely no financial documentation? Analysts chart stocks. They prepare these charts and make future projections based on recorded data. If you are going to succeed in the weight-loss business, you, too, must document your progress. You could also put the data in a Palm Pilot, digital diary, or computer. It is a great motivator to see in black and white that your exercises, the training poundage or resistance, the number of repetitions, the number of sets, the reduction in speed while performing the exercises, and your stability are all improving.

Sometimes, when clients feel they are in a rut and not improving with an exercise, I flip back a few pages on their program record to the weight at which they previously performed the exercise, show them the program card, and say, "Do you believe that three months ago you did this set with this weight?" They are always shocked and insist on seeing the old program page. This motivates them to continue, as they see what they have accomplished. The same will happen to you. So document.

The following is an example of a sample diary entry for cardiovascular exercise. Remember your exercise allocation, 25 percent cardiovascular and 75 percent strength and resistance training.

SAMPLE CARDIOVASCULAR EXERCISE DIARY

DATE	EXERCISE	TIME	INTENSITY	HEART RATE
1/1	Stationary Bike	15 minutes	Level 3	135–140
1/3	StairMaster	15 minutes	Level 4	140–145
1/5	Elliptical Trainer	5 minutes	Level 6	130–135
	Incline Treadmill	10 minutes	3.5 mph 4% Incline	140–145

This example provides an illustration of cross-training the cardiovascular portion of your exercise session by incorporating various activities spread among several days. The last entry illustrates that you may elect to perform two or more activities

133

during your cardiovascular portion. Remember, you are only going to allocate 25 percent of your exercise hour to cardiovascular activities.

SAMPLE STRENGTH AND RESISTANCE EXERCISE DIARY

DATE	EXERCISE	WEIGHT/BAND	REPETITIONS	SPEED
1/1	Lat Pulldown	Red Tube	12	4 counts down, 2 up
1/1	Rear Deltoid Fly	Green Tube	12	4 counts up, 2 down
1/1	Hip Extension	Green Tube	15	2 counts out, 2 back

Don't be afraid to be very detailed. The more specific you are, the more you will benefit. If the exercise terminology appears foreign, read on, as I will go into detail and provide a picture for each of the above exercises. I included this sample primarily to provide you with an example of diary entries.

5. PURCHASING

As with any start-up business, there will be capital expenditures. If you can't purchase these items all at once, then buy what your budget will allow and add in the future. Ideally, you will invest in the following:

New Shoes. Buy brand-new exercise shoes. Don't get an ancient pair out of the closet that you have had since the late eighties, when you last attempted an exercise program. They may look relatively unused, but believe me, the support structure has been weakened. Start fresh. Your body will thank you. You need the structure, cushioning, and support of a good, new pair of shoes, and plan to change them every three to four months (no, I don't own stock in shoe companies, which I have been accused of by clients in the past). Only use these shoes for exercise. Remember, the body's alignment starts at the feet. Take care of them. A good pair of shoes should cost you no more than seventy to eighty dollars. I don't personally care for cross-training shoes, since I don't believe in the concept of one shoe filling all needs. I do like running shoes, since I find they have the most support. The choice is yours. When you do go to the store, don't buy the first pair

EXERCISE SHOES SHOULD ONLY BE WORN DURING EXERCISE

The Business Plan for the Body

you try on. Try half a dozen. Certain brands and models fit quite differently. I happen to love New Balance shoes because they come in various widths and provide a good deal of support, but that is a personal preference.

And once again, these shoes are only for exercise. Don't wear them to the mall or to walk the dog. Only wear them for exercise.

A Heart Rate Monitor. As we discussed in Chapter 5, one of the best equipment investments you can make is a heart rate monitor. This monitor, worn every time you exercise, will give you invaluable information about how your body is responding to exercise. Heart rate monitors are approximately eighty dollars.

Exercise Equipment. The following equipment is also necessary for the successful execution of my recommended exercise plan:

Exercise tubing. Spri sells exercise tubing with handles and an attachment that will fit on an ordinary door. This tubing resembles a garden hose, only thinner, and comes in various color-coded tensions, with the handles attached at either end. This tubing is predominantly used for the upper body. Spri also manufactures exercise circles which, when placed around the legs, provide great resistance for working the lower body and also come in a variety of color-coded tensions. An additional benefit, these tubes and circles are perfect for taking your program on the road since they take up very little room in a suitcase. The cost is approximately seventy dollars for four bands and two circles.

Resist-a-ball. This large inflatable ball resembles a beach ball. It is used for a variety of exercises and places emphasis on the core of your body, which includes your abdominals and lower back. It is also great for creating instability, which, as I mentioned before, is an important element of progression. It costs approximately thirty to forty dollars, depending on the size.

Free weights in various sizes. Approximately fifty cents a pound. Starting with a pair of three-, five-, eight-, ten-, twelve-, and fifteen-pound weights is enough to get you started.

You can obtain additional information or purchase those products and others at my website, *www.businessplanforthebody. com.* Now, the actual program.

THE BUSINESS PLAN FOR THE BODY EXERCISE PROGRAM

The following program is a twelve-week exercise plan. As you will see in the next chapter, after the initial twelve-week startup, you will progress and expand upon this program. Each of the following exercises will constitute your first strategic plan. Before I describe the exercises, let's talk about what I refer to as the "Exercise Posture" you will assume at all times and review proper breathing techniques.

EXERCISE POSTURE

1. When performing a standing exercise, the following position should be assumed:
   a. Feet should be shoulder-width apart
   b. Toes are pointed forward
   c. Knees are soft, never locked
   d. Pull in your abdominal muscles
   e. Shoulders are back
   f. Neck and upper shoulders (trapezius muscles) are relaxed
   g. Chin is forward and head is up

2. When performing a sitting exercise, the following posture should be assumed:
   a. Feet are firmly planted on the floor
   b. Toes are pointed forward
   c. Pull in your abdominal muscles
   d. Shoulders are back
   e. Neck and upper shoulders (trapezius muscles) are relaxed
   f. Chin is forward and head is up

3. When lying down performing an exercise, the following position should be assumed:
   a. Pull in your abdominal muscles

b. Shoulders are relaxed

c. Neck is neutral and in alignment with spine

BREATHING

I frequently observe individuals holding their breath when exercising. It is important to be aware of proper breathing, especially during strength and resistance exercises. As a general rule, exhale on the exertion, or the hard part of the exercise, and inhale as you release the tension on the muscle. In technical terms, this is called exhaling on the contraction, or as you squeeze the muscle, and inhaling as you release the tension on the muscle and return to starting position. I urge you to breathe slowly. Over the years, I have coached clients to inhale and exhale as if they have a straw in their mouth. This style of breathing will train you to take long, controlled breaths rather than short gulps of air that will not provide you with enough oxygen. Try these guidelines or modify them so you're comfortable with the process. Just make sure not to hold your breath during the exercises.

DON'T HOLD YOUR BREATH WHEN EXERCISING

STRENGTH AND RESISTANCE PROGRAM #1

1. Lat Pulldown—Back

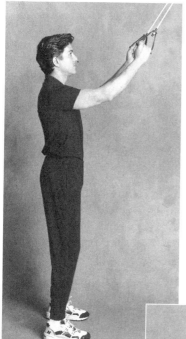

1. Attach the Spri Xertube to the top of a door using the Spri door attachment. The door attachment, which is a nylon strap with a loop at the end, fits at the top of any door and holds the tubing in place.
2. Adopt the standing position with palms facing forward in the tube's handles.
3. Slowly exhale as you pull your elbows down to your sides, inhale up.
4. Make sure to concentrate on your back muscles and squeeze, or contract the muscles, at the bottom portion of the movement.
5. Keep your shoulders and neck muscles relaxed at all times.

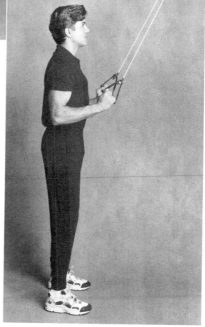

2. Back Row—Back

1. Attach the Spri Xertube using the door attachment on the side of a door.
2. Adopt the standing position with palms facing forward in the tube's handles.
3. Slowly exhale as you pull your elbows to your sides, inhale as you release.
4. Make sure to concentrate on your back muscles and squeeze, or contract the muscles, as you pull back.
5. Keep your shoulders and neck muscles relaxed at all times.

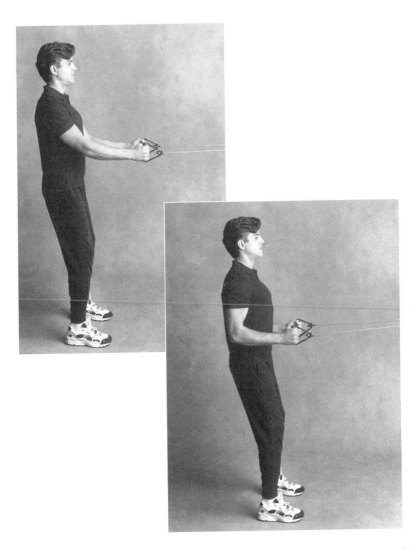

Preservation of Capital

3. Rear Deltoid Fly—Rear Portion of the Shoulder

1. Wrap the Spri Xertube using the door attachment on the side of a door at chest height.
2. Adopt the standing position with palms facing forward in the tube's handles.
3. Slowly exhale as you pull your hands out to your sides, inhale as you return.
4. Make sure to keep your elbows only slightly bent.
5. Concentrate on the back of your shoulders, the rear deltoids, as you pull.
6. Keep your shoulders and neck muscles relaxed at all times.

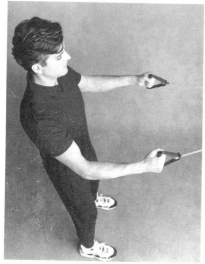

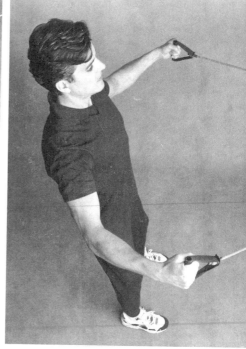

The Business Plan for the Body

4. Standing Lateral Raise—Middle Portion of the Shoulder

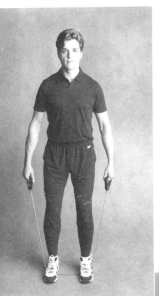

1. Place the yellow or green Spri Xertube under your feet.
2. Adopt the standing position on top of the band with palms facing in.
3. Slightly lean forward to isolate the medial, or middle part, of the shoulder.
4. Slowly exhale as you lift the tube up to your sides to shoulder height, inhale down.
5. Make sure to keep your elbows only slightly bent.
6. Make sure to concentrate on the middle of your shoulders, the medial deltoids, as you lift the band.
7. Keep your shoulders and neck muscles relaxed at all times

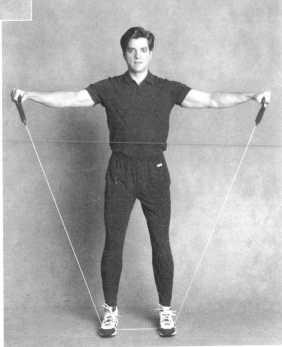

5. Push-up—Chest and Tricep

1. Place your hands shoulder-width apart, fingers spread.
2. If you are a beginner, balance on your knees. If you feel stronger, lift up on your toes.
3. Keep your abdominals tucked at all times to support your lower back.
4. Slowly inhale as you lower down to two inches above the floor, exhale as you press back up.
5. Make sure your chin goes just over your fingertips.
6. Concentrate on your chest at all times, especially as you press up.
7. If you fatigue early on your toes, then drop down to your knees to complete the set of repetitions.

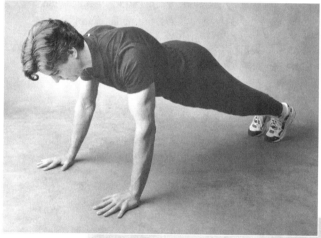

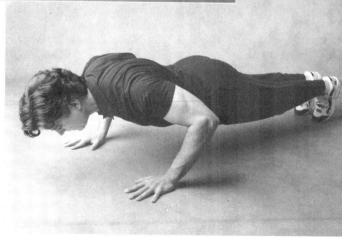

6. Tricep Push-down—Tricep

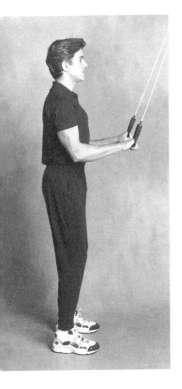

1. Attach the Spri Xertube to the top of a door, using the Spri door attachment.
2. Adopt the standing position, elbows at your sides, with palms facing down in the tube's handles.
3. Slowly exhale as you press your hands down to your sides, inhale up.
4. Make sure to concentrate on the back of your arms, the triceps, and squeeze, or contract the muscles at the bottom portion of the movement.
5. Keep your shoulders and neck muscles relaxed at all times.

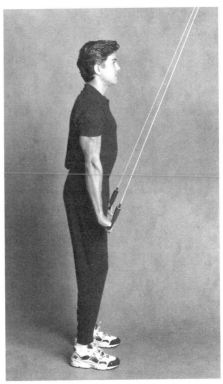

7. Bicep Curl Sitting on the Ball—Bicep

1. Assume the sitting position with light weights to begin in each hand.
2. Slowly exhale as you lift the weights with palms facing up, inhale down.
3. Concentrate on your biceps as you lift and slowly release.
4. Make sure not to swing the dumbbells. Move slowly through each repetition.
5. Keep your elbows at your sides. Don't allow them to lift up.

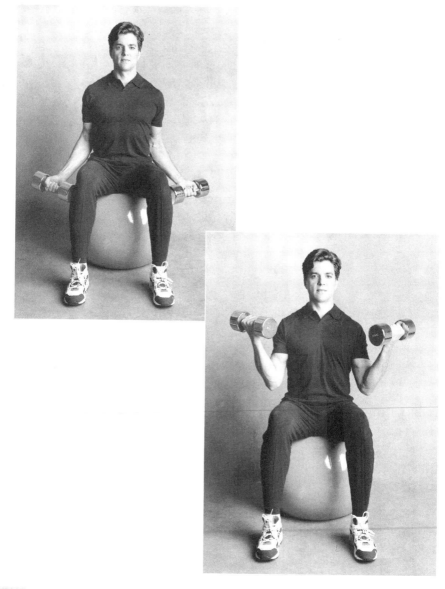

8. Squats—Lower Body

1. Adopt the standing position with the toes pointing forward, abdominals tucked and shoulders back.
2. Slowly inhale as you squat down until your hamstrings, the back of your legs, are parallel with the floor.
3. Exhale as you press through your heels and concentrate on squeezing your gluts, your rear end, as you lift.
4. Don't let your knees go beyond your toes. If they do, then you need to sit farther back.

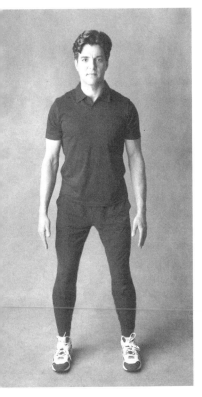

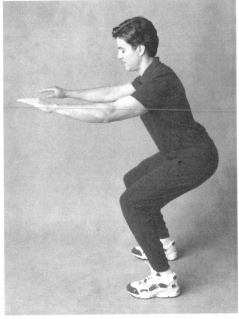

9. Stationary Lunges—Lower Body

1. Place your right foot forward, left foot back.
2. Toes face forward with weight evenly distributed between both legs.
3. Slowly inhale as you lower your body, bending both knees. Hold, then exhale as you slowly lift up to starting position.
4. Concentrate on your gluts, your rear end, throughout the exercise.
5. Keep your abdominals tucked at all times. Don't lean forward.
6. Make sure your forward knee does not pass your forward toe. If it does, then you need to spread your legs farther apart.
7. Repeat the exercise on the other leg.

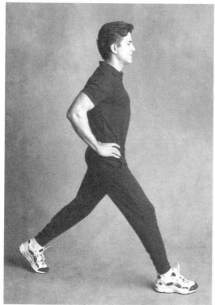

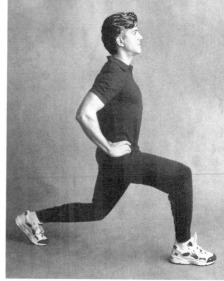

10. Hamstring Curl on the Ball—Hamstring

1. Lie down on your back with your heels on the ball.
2. Make sure your abdominals are tucked and your neck is relaxed.
3. Slowly exhale as you pull your heels to your lower back. The ball will move toward you.
4. Hold at the end point, squeeze your hamstrings, then release and inhale.
5. Make sure to keep your legs in alignment at all times.

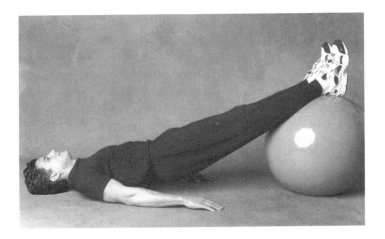

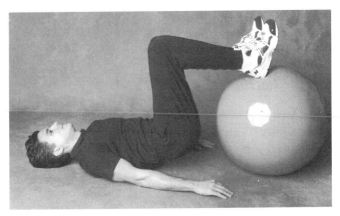

Preservation of Capital

11. Hip Extension—Gluteus Maximus and Hamstring

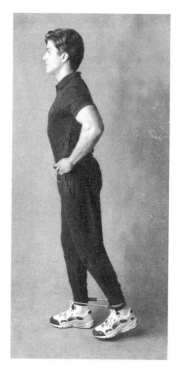

1. Place the green Spri Xering around your ankles.
2. Adopt the standing position with the left foot slightly bent and the right leg straight.
3. Slowly exhale as you press the right leg back, pause, then inhale as you release.
4. Once you begin the movement, keep constant tension on the muscle at all times.
5. Make sure to concentrate on your gluts as you squeeze the leg back.
6. Don't be surprised if you feel a slight burn in both the right and left gluteus maximus. The left leg will be challenged as it is used to support your body weight.
7. Repeat the exercise on the other leg.

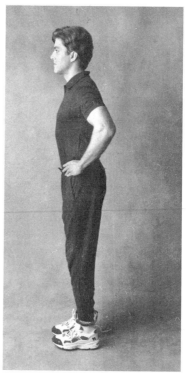

The Business Plan for the Body

12. Hip Abduction—Outer Thigh, the Abductor Muscle, and Gluteus Maximus

1. Place the green Spri Xering around your ankles.
2. Adopt the standing position with the left foot slightly bent and the right leg straight.
3. Slowly exhale as you press the right leg out to your side, pause, then inhale as you return.
4. Once you begin the movement, keep constant tension on the muscle at all times.
5. Make sure to concentrate on your outer thigh as you squeeze the leg out.
6. Don't be surprised if you feel a slight burn in both the left and the right gluteus maximus, or both sides of your rear end. The left leg and glut will be challenged, as it is used to support your body weight.
7. Repeat the exercise on the other leg.

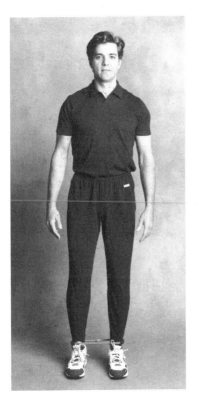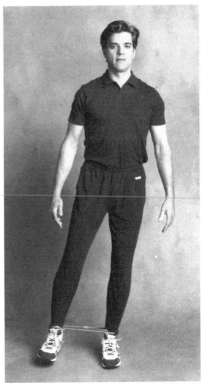

13. Back Extension—Lower Back

1. Position yourself on your hands and knees with a flat back.
2. Your arms and legs should be shoulder-width apart.
3. Slowly exhale as you lift the left arm and right leg up simultaneously. Hold, then repeat on the other side.
4. Keep your chin down and your abdominals tucked at all times.
5. Concentrate on your back at all times as you lift and release.

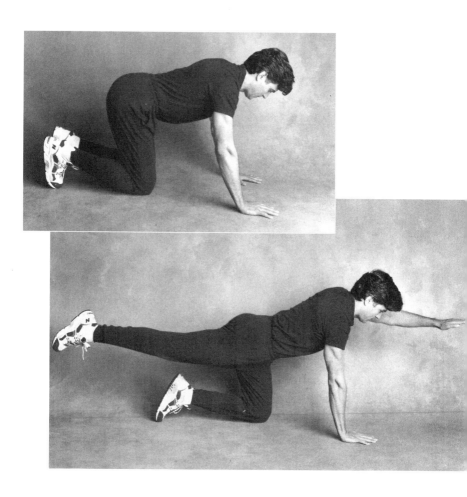

The Business Plan for the Body

14. Bridging on the Ball—Lower Back

1. Lie down on the ball with your head and shoulders supported on the ball.
2. Place your feet in front of you, shoulder-width apart with toes forward.
3. Start with your gluteus maximus (rear end) relaxed and lower than your chest.
4. Slowly exhale as you lift your gluteus maximus and lower back, inhale as you release. Your abdominals and legs should end parallel with the floor.
5. As you lift, concentrate on squeezing your gluteus maximus and lower back.

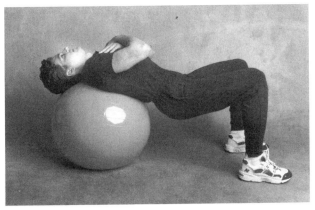

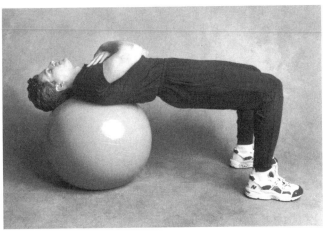

15. Abdominals

1. Sit on the ball with feet shoulder-width apart, toes forward.
2. Slightly lean back, placing tension on your abdominals.
3. Slowly exhale as you lift up about three inches, then lower and inhale.
4. Concentrate at all times on your abdominals. If you feel pain in your back, stop.
5. Make sure to keep your chin in alignment at all times.

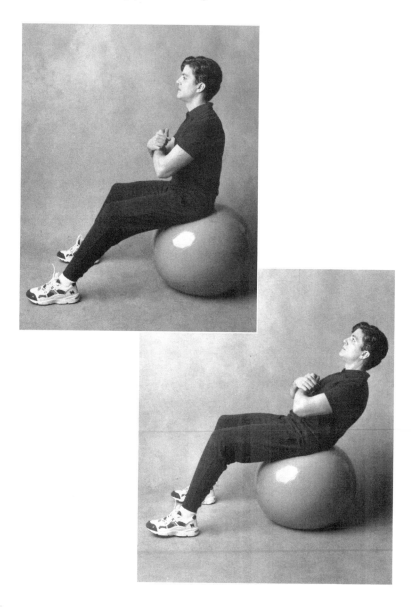

The Business Plan for the Body

In executing your program, each time you perform these exercises you should plan to complete one set of twelve to fifteen repetitions. When you are able to complete fifteen repetitions with ease, then you must progress your program, which we discuss in Chapter 9. With your cardiovascular warm-up and one set of each exercise, plan between forty-five minutes and one hour for each workout. Commit to at least two workouts per week, ideally three or more, and stick with it.

If you will be exercising in a health club, building exercise facility, park district, or some other environment where you may have access to a variety of equipment, use it. I by no means feel that exercising with free weights and tubing, as my program pictured, is the only option. I use a little bit of everything in my personal program. Use the equipment available to you, supplement when necessary, and just remember to devote two-thirds of your time to the back of the body and one-third to the front. The program I gave you can be used when traveling, or in your home or office.

COMPLETE ONE SET OF 12 TO 15 REPETITIONS, THEN PROGRESS

My exercise program does place an emphasis on the back of the body. As previously mentioned in this chapter, one of the big buzzwords in exercise right now relates to the "structural integrity" of the body. Basically, structural integrity means that the body is in alignment. So often, we hear or have personally experienced an injury, tennis elbow, bad knees, rotator cuff tear, bulging cervical disk, bad back, etc. What do those terms mean? They indicate that there is an imbalance, or integrity problem, within the body. As discussed earlier, a great many of these problems stem from muscular imbalance. In life, we generally use the front of the body more frequently than the back. As an example, get up from a chair. You just used your quadriceps, or the front of your legs. Now go climb a staircase. Once again, you used the front of your legs. When do you use the back of the legs or hamstring muscles? Not nearly as frequently. The same applies to your upper body. Every time you carry a grocery bag, a child, or a box, you use the front of the body, including the chest and front of the shoulder (anterior deltoid). Unless you regularly row boats or ride horses, you never use your back muscles (latisimus dorsi, rhomboids, and low mid-trapezius muscles). That is why these muscles need to be strengthened through exercise. Some of these problems relate to our genetic alignment, such as a

153

curvature of the spine, but others are more likely because of the way we live and carry ourselves on a daily basis.

Consider how cars, television, and computers have affected our lives. We spend a countless amount of time sitting in the car or hunched over our desks or computers. Aside from this being one of the primary reasons for this country's current obesity epidemic, it has additionally led to a dramatic rise in problems related to muscular imbalance. Examine your posture as you are reading this book. Are your shoulders rounded? Probably. Is your neck jutting forward? Most likely. Is your lower back rounded? The chances are great that it is. Are you propped up in bed? Maybe. Sitting in a very cushy chair? Are you eating? (Just kidding.) These are the positions and postures that can contribute to alignment problems in the future. Remember, being overweight additionally affects body alignment since you are forcing the body to carry an increased amount of weight on its frame. Once again, the human body does not want to be overweight, nor was it designed to be.

Therefore, my exercise program focuses on the back of the body and the strengthening of those particular muscles. Again, face a mirror. Are your shoulders rounded? Stand to the side. Is the front part of your leg far more developed than the back? These are the imbalances strength and resistance training will correct, both visually and structurally. So think of this strength and resistance program as not only helping you to enhance your posture, look better, and lose weight, but also to balance your body and keep you pain and injury free.

STRATEGIC ACTION PLAN

You have made a decision to preserve capital, in this case lean muscle tissue, and profit from your endeavors. You have decided to make exercise a priority, as you realize exercise is an essential component in the weight-loss business. You have been given an exercise prescription to lose weight. It's a different prescription than you've attempted or heard of in the past because now you will devote 25 percent of your exercise time to cardiovascular exercise and 75 percent to strength and resistance training. If you are dubious about this prescription, I ask you to again recall the anecdote that began this chapter. Observe the appearances of those who spend hours on cardiovascular work and those who employ predominantly strength and resistance training programs. Who appears to be the more successful in the weight-loss business? We have examined the misconceptions surrounding strength and resistance training. You have done the strategic planning to schedule two to three hours a week for your workouts. You are going to allocate two-thirds of your strength and resistance program to the back of the body and one-third to the front of the body to improve your posture and the body's "structural integrity." You are purchasing new exercise shoes, a heart rate monitor, and the simple inexpensive equipment I recommended. Prior to investing in exercise, you will assess your weaknesses, strengthen those you identify, and document your progress. You will be the man with a plan, an exercise plan that will yield terrific profits for years to come.

Unlike so many other investment opportunities, there are few risks with this plan. Therefore, you've just made an extremely wise investment decision. Alan Greenspan will not stall your plan. Russian economic woes will not cause you to stray from your plan. A sudden downturn in the Asian market or the collapse of high-technology stocks—none of these can prevent you from achieving your goal. Unlike the investment marketplace, only one person is responsible for the success of your investment plan—you. You are creating a controlled investment environment. You aren't looking for a "quick fix."

YOUR ARE THE CEO OF YOUR BODY

You are investing for the future. Unlike an investment in a hot stock that might yield huge returns for a brief period of time, you can make an investment in your body that yields benefits for the rest of your life. Though no one can predict what the years may bring, keep in mind that your body, your health, and your appearance will profit since you committed to *The Business Plan for the Body.*

ESTABLISHING REALISTIC INVESTMENT GOALS

8 *You Were Patient Putting It On, Be Patient Taking It Off*

"Patience is power. With time and patience the mulberry leaf becomes silk."

CHINESE PROVERB

Remember, I told you about a program my firm provides in Chicago that's called the "Ten, Ten, Ten Plan." For $10,000 we fitness-train clients for ten hours a week for ten weeks and guarantee that they will lose ten pounds. If they don't lose a minimum of ten pounds, we refund their money. I speak with the participants of this program each day and plan all their meals, whether those meals be at home, at a restaurant, or at an event. To this day, all participants have lost at least ten pounds, some as much as twenty-six pounds. One of our clients, "Alicia," lost twenty-one and three-quarter pounds in ten weeks. She accomplished this by doing the following:

- Fitness-trained for ten hours every week. She only missed one hour one week because of illness.
- She never ate more than 1,000 calories a day.
- She drank tons of water.

What is my point? Simple. She lost approximately two pounds a week eating 1,000 calories a day and fitness-training ten hours a week. How, I ask, can certain programs claim that you can lose five, ten, even fifteen pounds a week and have it be real weight loss? That answer is equally simple. THEY CAN'T. Granted, even Alicia's program was rather drastic. It is usually employed by people who want quick results, and keep in mind that quick

*results mean two pounds a week. That's two pounds a week,
not some ridiculous tabloid teaser "Lose Ten Pounds in Ten
Minutes!"*

I want to revisit your present situation. You decided to go
into the weight-loss business. You looked at the competition,
then you went public and assembled your management team.
Next, you examined the "financials." You proceeded to explore
intelligent eating strategies and formulated a result-producing
exercise prescription. What's next? Simple, the establishment of
realistic, achievable "investment" goals.

Traditionally, investors assign a valuation to a publicly
traded stock. Investors look at market share, management performance, the product offering and/or services, marketing
plan, and other relevant data. Most of all they review the
financials looking for an increase in profits coupled with consistently met earnings projections. Consider the following
example. Americans love market gurus such as Warren Buffett
and his holding company, Berkshire Hathaway. Buffett is
a classic long-term investor, never a short-term
trader, who sets realistic goals and rarely if ever
disappoints. To be called a "Buffett" investor
would be the equivalent of saying someone is
intelligent, well-researched, and, above all, realistic with regard to his or her expectations and
long-term goals. That is the kind of program I am
creating for you. Haven't we all lost money trying to make a
quick dollar? We trade a stock or option, simply on supposed
"inside" information from a friend; a broker convinces us the
company is the next Netscape; or we think we have all the
information to make fast money. Be honest, how many times
has this translated into a successful stock pick for you? I personally could go on for hours about my "bad" stock trades. No
more. I now make intelligent investment decisions based on
diligent research and long-term projections. I am requiring
you to do the same with your weight-loss projections, what I
term "Managing Expectations."

Expectations play a significant role in the valuation of stocks.
When expectations are not met, invariably investors and share-
holders become angry and they punish the stock by selling it.
What happened? Did the company actually stumble or did it set

**BECOME A "BUF-
FETT" INVESTOR—
SET REALISTIC
GOALS**

unrealistically high earning expectations that were virtually impossible to achieve?

My belief is that most individuals attempting to lose weight set unrealistic goals. Why? There are several reasons, not the least of which is the mass media. Day after day, week after week, I see a tabloid headline, a magazine cover, a television infomercial, or a talk show go on and on about quick weight loss. I have recently seen the same advertisement that states "Lose up to 10 lbs. this weekend! The Hollywood 'Miracle' diet features delicious, all-natural juices that help you lose weight while you cleanse, detoxify, and rejuvenate your body." This clearly is impossible. In the same vein, the cover of another national publication screamed "Lose as Much as You Want, 10, 20, 30 Pounds with No Effort." With no effort? I don't think so. As we have established, Americans are in the midst of a full-blown obesity epidemic. Consequently, a lot of desperate people are seeking a solution. Unfortunately, the solution to weight loss is not quick. Weight loss requires effort, time, and discipline, as does financial investing. Remember in my analysis of the competition in Chapter 2, anything that includes the words "quick" and "weight loss" together is false. It doesn't happen, and to state it does is highly irresponsible.

Be honest with me and yourself. Did you gain the excess weight in a day, a week, or a month? No. You and I know that it took time to gain weight. According to the National Center for Health Statistics, the average American puts on ten pounds each decade. That's the *average* American; many gain considerably more. You want to reverse that trend. How can you possibly think that going on a diet for a few days or a few weeks is going to shed pounds that took months, years, maybe decades to accumulate?

Fact: We know that 3,500 calories equals one pound. Therefore, can it be possible to lose ten pounds in ten days? That would mean expending 35,000 more calories in ten days than you consumed during that time period. Is this possible? Yes, but highly unlikely. Think about marathon runners. During most marathons the average-size runner burns approximately 3,500 calories, which is equal to one pound. Now, for those of you who have never run a marathon and don't know anyone who has, most runners make sure to consume as many calories

The Business Plan for the Body

as they burn for peak performance. For the sake of argument, assume that they don't. If you were to run a marathon, fifty kilometers or 26.2 miles a day for *ten* consecutive days, then maybe, and I mean maybe, you might lose ten pounds in ten days, but most certainly your feet, knees, lower back, immune system, and most everything else would be injured or severely impaired before you could complete this task.

Another possible way to lose ten pounds in ten days would be to fast. We know from Chapter 2 that fasting is by no means recommended, nor is it a key to permanent weight loss. Fasting places the body in ketosis, similar to what a high-protein diet achieves, which is a toxic state for the body. It also severely diminishes your basal metabolic rate.

What most "quick fix" diets do is affect your water weight and lean muscle tissue. Let's start with lean muscle tissue. We know, from the preceding chapter, that lean muscle is the body's most active tissue, and similar to capital in an investment program, it must be preserved. Don't forget, muscles are the "big spenders" and burn lots of calories twenty-four hours a day. Most severely restrictive diets trick the body into believing that it is on a deserted island with minimal or no food. Therefore, as a defense mechanism, the body attacks its most active tissue, muscle, in order to slow down the body's basal metabolic rate. As previously established, muscle is the body's most metabolically active tissue. Therefore, by attacking muscle, the body will burn fewer calories each day and stay alive longer. This is exactly what you do *not* want to do.

The second phenomenon that occurs during a restrictive diet is loss of water. As you severely restrict calories, you lose some of the bloat you have been carrying around for months, possibly years. How? First, when you are dehydrated, as most individuals are when they begin a diet, your body perceives that there is not a readily available source of water. So the body holds on to its remaining water supply in the outer tissues of the body. You puff up. On a restrictive diet that urges you to drink lots of water (since the creators of the diet know that you will then lose water weight) the scale goes down as the body releases the reserves of water as it is properly hydrated. Second, you also drastically reduce your sodium content on most restrictive diets, which contributes to the bloat. This will also produce water loss. Third, as this especially applies to high-protein, low-carbohydrate diets, when you first stop eating carbohydrates, your body reacts by releasing water that's stored with your body's supply of carbohydrates. Therefore, most of the weight loss is water, not fat. After three or four days you jump on the scale and say, "Hey, I lost five pounds!" Did you really lose five pounds? No, you lost four pounds of water weight you have been carrying around and one pound of body fat. The moment you return to your old eating habits, the water weight will come right back on.

This has happened hundreds of times when my clients go to health spas. Now please, don't misunderstand, there is nothing wrong with a spa. It can actually be a great way to jump-start a weight-loss program. But here is a phenomenon I constantly observe. A client goes to a spa and loses seven pounds in five days. This is what occurs. At the spa, they ply you with water and foods with high water counts such as fruits and vegetables. Consequently, you lost about three to four pounds of water bloat. Because you were eating primarily fruits and vegetables, you also lost a few pounds of waste from your colon. What amount of body fat did you actually lose? Probably, at most, two pounds. Then you got on a plane to come home. You had a drink, ate peanuts, and the plane food, which is loaded with sodium, and flew in a pressurized cabin, which is very dehydrating. The next day you got on your scale at home and screamed, "What, I've gained five pounds back?" Did you really gain five pounds in a day? No. Did you put back the five pounds of bloat and colon buildup? Yes.

Look at this cycle. Say you go on a crazy seven-day diet. The scale does go down, but is it body fat, muscle, or water that you lost? Only with a slow weight-loss protocol can we be reasonably sure that you are losing body fat. Why? For the sake of this discussion, let's assume you are in perfect water balance—you drink between 80 to 100 ounces of water each day and your urine is clear, an indication that you are well-hydrated. This indicates the weight loss is not water. Let's also assume that you are strength and resistance training and your training poundage, or the amount of weight you are able to lift, remains current or increases. This would indicate that you are not losing muscle. Then, when the scale goes down, we know that you are losing body fat, not muscle or water.

WHAT IS A REALISTIC WEIGHT-LOSS GOAL?

Instead of randomly picking a number, which most of us do when we attempt weight loss, let's be smart, use the new knowledge we have, and revisit the numbers. Go back to the equation we explored in Chapter 5 dealing with basal metabolic rate (BMR). What was the number you came up with? Since I previously used myself as an example, let's use those numbers once again. If you recall, we determined that my total caloric output each day was 2,875. Therefore, in a given week, if I average 2,875 calories each day, I will maintain my weight. If I ate 500 fewer calories on average each day, at the end of a week, or seven times 500 calories, I would lose 3,500 calories, or one pound. If I wanted to lose two pounds in a week, I would have to eat 1,000 fewer calories on average each day. You get the idea. But wait, I only approached weight loss from one side of the equation, the calories in. What about the calories out?

REVISIT THE NUMBERS

Yes, as we also established in Chapter 5, you can rev up your metabolism through exercise, specifically by focusing on strength and resistance exercises. So, going back to your equation, you can increase the number of calories you burn each day through exercise. Get out your calculator and see how your numbers will dramatically increase using a more active multiplier.

Personally, I can't approach weight loss through additional exercise. I already allocate five hours a week to my program and I feel that is enough. As part of my five hours, I do a fifteen-minute-plus cardiovascular warm-up followed by aggressive strength training. I know people who allocate more time to weight loss, but for me, I have established, both physically and emotionally, that five hours is enough. You probably are not at five hours a week of exercise, so you can easily increase your multiplier through effective, additional exercise. Remember, the effective exercise prescription is 25 percent cardiovascular and 75 percent strength and resistance training.

Can you lose ten pounds in ten days? Not really. Can you lose from one-half to two pounds a week? Yes. Now, I don't mean to give the female population a hard time, but it is true that men

Establishing Realistic Investment Goals

will lose weight faster than most women, given the same caloric intake, because they are larger, generally more muscular, and therefore burn more calories. If a man and a woman went on a similar program, ate the same number of calories, and exercised with similar frequency, intensity, and duration, the man would lose more weight simply because he is creating a larger caloric deficit. Look at this chart:

REALISTIC WEIGHT-LOSS EXPECTATIONS FOR MEN AND WOMEN

	MAN	WOMAN
Calories to Maintain Weight	2,900	1,900
Calories Consumed Each Day	1,500	1,500
Caloric Deficit Each Day	1,400	400
Total Deficit for One Week (Multiply Daily Deficit by 7 days)	9,800	2,800
Total Pounds Lost for One Week (Divide Weekly Deficit by 3,500 calories)	2.8	0.8

If you are a woman, please don't be discouraged by these figures. Instead, remember this: The key to weight loss is the creation of a caloric deficit. For years I have said to clients, "If you aren't losing weight, you aren't creating a caloric deficit." Remember, *calories in minus calories out determines your body weight.* At the present, you have established the perfect equation to be at your current weight. This is something you must understand. You *created* your present weight. Now we will change that equation in order for you to lose weight.

UNREALISTIC EXPECTATIONS WILL ONLY LEAD TO FAILURE

I introduced the concept of "managing expectations" earlier in this chapter. By that expression I mean you have to establish goals that can be attained. If you set too high an expectation in your weight-loss plan and it is not met, you will be discouraged and likely feel you failed. The same holds true for investors in a stock when that corporation misses its earning's projection. The shareholders may be discouraged and consider selling their holding. In other words, neither the company nor you have realistically managed your expectations. According to Thomas Wadden, an obesity expert at the University of Pennsylvania, "satisfaction is comparing what you expect and what you get.

The Business Plan for the Body

If you keep ratcheting up your expectations, you'll get dissatisfied and quit." Think about this for a moment and see if it applies to you. You finally decide to try to lose weight. You embrace some "program" that you read about or heard someone discussing on a radio or television show, and you attempt to lose weight. Don't forget, I know about this pattern. I did the same thing for years. So, you're on some diet, you feel deprived, maybe a little irritable, and hungry. Then you get on the scale. "What! That's all I lost!" You ditch the program and make a beeline to the House of Pies.

This is behaving the way impatient investors do when they hear any bit of negative news about a stock. They bail. Was this a wise investment decision? Not if the fundamentals are still in place and your investment program is on track.

Where was the error? The error lies in your unrealistic expectations of weight loss. Had you set a more attainable weight-loss goal, you would most likely still be on plan. This time will be different. You will plug in the numbers. You will be informed. You will proceed intelligently. You've established realistic, attainable goals.

You possess the power to determine the speed at which you desire to lose weight. If you want to be aggressive on your plan, then cut back on your calories and make sure to get in five hours a week of exercise. Remember our client Alicia who lost two pounds a week by eating 1,000 calories a day and exercising ten hours a week with a professional fitness trainer. That is aggressive weight loss. If you want to ease yourself into the plan, then set a more conservative goal and be pleased when you see the scale respond. In addition, as you are setting goals, take a good look at your life. What can you realistically devote in money, time, energy, and emotion to your plan?

YOU CONTROL THE SPEED AT WHICH YOU LOSE WEIGHT

First, examine the financial aspects involved. Consider these factors. You might have to join a health club or purchase home exercise equipment. I outlined the basic equipment you will need to buy in the purchasing section of Chapter 7, but additional equipment may be needed as you progress your program. If it is necessary to ease yourself into your plan because of the expense, don't worry. Similar to a savings plan or investment program where you allocate a certain amount of monthly income, over time, with interest and growth, your investment will grow. The same applies as you allocate more dollars to your "plan" because, ultimately, it will enhance your investment.

Second, review the time involved. How will you fit exercise into what I will assume is a full schedule? I can't tell you how many times I meet with a prospective client who says, "I hate getting up early but I am going to give it a try. So schedule me for Monday, Wednesday, and Friday at 6:00 A.M." I always discourage this strategy. Think about it. You hate getting up, probably have a similar feeling regarding exercise, so you are going to punish yourself by doing both? Not smart. I promise you, you will quit. Decide on an exercise time that fits better into your lifestyle and personal needs. If you are presently not exercising and you plan to exercise even once in the next week, then I say great. You are trying. Maybe soon you will go to twice a week, then three times. Do you see a pattern here? There is nothing wrong with easing oneself into the program. The key is consistency.

CONSISTENCY IS THE KEY

Third, look at your physical energy. Going "on plan" takes energy. You will have to think about your food, do research to increase your "caloric awareness," and find not just the time, but the energy, to exercise. Make a wise projection and trust your instincts. Prioritize. You might eliminate some current activities to make time for your new venture, the weight-loss business. We only have so much physical energy to draw upon on a daily basis. Similar to your caloric allocation, we all devise an energy allocation for ourselves. Energy is a commodity. Energy needs to be preserved, similar to our plan's capital—muscle. Fact: The more you sleep, within reason, the more energy you will have, so examine your sleep patterns and try to improve upon them if need be. Don't plan other strenuous activities, such as mowing the lawn, cleaning, or "power shopping" on the days you plan to exercise. Map out a week in advance if you find it helpful. Plan, don't leave things to chance.

LEARN TO PRIORITIZE

Fourth, assess your mental health. I know this might sound funny, but you have to take a moment to evaluate your mental state and how ready you are to meet the demands of the plan. You must realize that going into the weight-loss business is

The Business Plan for the Body

going to require inner strength and discipline, just as any investment does. If this is a stress-filled time in your life and you are feeling low, then don't overreach in your weight-loss expectations. Make this a positive in your life, not a negative.

Consider your emotional relationship to food. Many of us use food as emotional comfort. We use food when we feel anxious, stressed, upset, or even bored. In these instances, we generally turn to comfort foods, carbohydrates such as cookies, pie, cakes, mashed potatoes, chips or pasta, all of which are high in calories, sugar, or fat. I earlier mentioned that eating carbohydrates stimulates the production of serotonin, which is a brain chemical that regulates mood. Many medically prescribed antidepressants stimulate the production of serotonin, consequently, eating carbohydrates is similar to self-medicating oneself to enhance your mood and make you feel better.

Realistically assess the time you can devote to exercise each week. Review your schedule and fit exercise in when it makes sense. Don't just say, "I am going to exercise every day for two hours," when you know that will never happen. You will just be setting yourself up to fail. So be honest.

This process of establishing realistic goals will necessitate you reviewing your plan to date. First of all, it takes courage to say, "I am going to succeed at weight loss." You probably have not succeeded in the past. But don't forget, this time you have a plan. This time you did the necessary research. This time you worked "the numbers." So, give yourself a break, trust your ability, and forge ahead toward your goal.

AS YOU ARE SETTING PROJECTIONS, KEEP THESE POINTS IN MIND

Never eat less than 1,000 calories a day. Eating less than that amount could place your body in starvation mode, which we addressed earlier, and slow your metabolism. This is not the goal. The goal is to increase your metabolism. In addition, who can realistically stay on a plan of less than 1,000 calories a day? It is totally unrealistic and goes against everything I have addressed in this chapter. Though I did use my client Alicia as an example of someone who did stay on this 1,000-calorie plan, it's tough to do and not the way we eat in "real life."

Don't skip meals. We talked about this in Chapter 6. Skipping meals could slow your metabolism or lead you to binge at the next meal. No skipping.

Don't overexercise. Alicia, on our ten-week program, exercised ten hours a week. But she did so with a professional fitness trainer who made sure her joints, back, neck, etc., were not overstressed. She was in a safe environment. Ten hours a week is aggressive, but her expectations were high and ultimately met.

Don't exercise to eat. Please, don't undertake an exercise program simply to justify overeating. Over time, excessive eating will most likely require you to add even more exercise. So you end up overeating and overexercising. This "plan" will likely lead to injury from overuse, such as a bad back or bad knees. Once injured, you will gain weight as you continue to eat with fervor while not expending those excess calories through exercise.

As a smart businessperson, before you begin to establish goals, you need to assess your current "financial" situation. I want you to use the following criteria to assess your present condition and your progress:

Get on the scale. As I mentioned in Chapter 2, most people have absolutely no idea how much they weigh. I don't care what kind of a scale you use, though I personally like the balance beam scales similar to those in doctors' offices. Once you have weighed yourself, this is the *only* scale you will weigh yourself on. You are forbidden to jump on a scale at your friend's house, or at a hotel, or anywhere else. One scale. Consistent data. You should weigh yourself *once* a week, same day, same time. Record your weight on a weekly basis in your food diary/exercise journal. This way you keep all the records of your progress in one place.

I personally weigh myself every Monday morning. If my weight is up, I proclaim, "This week, Cycle 3." Do you remember the dog food manufacturer that made a special formula, Cycle 3, for overweight dogs? That's what I call my weight-loss program when my weight creeps up—Cycle 3.

Even my weight goes up from time to time. I am human. Sometimes I consume too many calories. I always exercise, so that is not an issue. It does help owning a firm of twelve personal fitness trainers, so I don't have a problem getting a trainer when I want one. But at times I know I do eat too much. Since I get on the scale every week, I am able to get the added weight off *immediately,* rather than letting it sit there. I quickly gather the data about myself.

That is what you have undoubtedly not done in the past. You ignored the weight gain. You hauled it around with you. You didn't get the data from the scale. You either believed the scale was incorrect or you embraced denial. Experts indicate that people who maintain weight loss hop on the scale at least once a week. You *must* do the same.

Similarly, don't weigh yourself constantly. It only leads to discouragement when your water weight fluctuates, as it does on a daily basis. I know countless investors who check their stocks ten times a day. They drive their brokers crazy, and those around them, with a barrage of calls every time their holding goes down one-eighth of a point, which is, after all, only twelve and one-half cents. Trust your long-term projections, and avoid the daily fluctuations that could sabotage your weight-loss investment plan.

A note of caution: When you first get on the scale, you may be shocked, but don't be discouraged. Instead of being disappointed in yourself for letting the situation get out of hand, applaud yourself for taking positive steps to correct the problem.

Take measurements. I like this concept because, especially with strength and resistance training, you will really see a positive change in these stats. Have a friend or family member do the basics: chest, waist, hips, individual thighs, and upper arms. Repeat these measurements approximately once a month, or every other month. Keep the data in your food diary/exercise journal or in your computer along with your weekly weight. Look at the trend and be pleased with the results.

Try on clothes. A client, Holly, has a great idea. She says I should tell each of my clients once a month to put on their favorite jeans, suit, and black tie outfit. I can't tell you how many black tie events I go to where the men look like hell in these twenty-five-year-old tuxedos they've squeezed themselves into. Do you remember the movie *Father of the Bride?* Spencer Tracy, or Steve Martin in the remake, have a hilarious scene where he is trying on his old tuxedo for his daughter's upcoming wedding. The buttons are straining to support his stomach and his pants are at least three inches too short.

Ultimately, he ends up splitting the seat of his pants. Sure it's funny, but it's also art imitating life.

But I do like the concept of using your old clothes as a gauge. It is inspirational to put something on that at one time was too tight and confining and have it once again fit. Keep in mind, when you bought the garment it was your size. Yes, you did once fit in these clothes. If you can once again comfortably wear them that's great—though it might be a good idea to update your look! Try it. See if it works for you. "Props" may provide just the stimuli you require to stay with your plan. Also, this may be the first time in a long time that your clothes are getting looser instead of tighter.

Let's review:

1. Weigh yourself once a week, same scale, same time, same day.
2. Take body measurements once a month or every other month.
3. Once a month, try on the same set of clothes. See the difference.

MEASURING BODY FAT

You may be thinking, "What about body fat? Why aren't we going to use that as an additional gauge?" At this point I'd like to briefly discuss body fat and the three most frequently used techniques employed to measure it. Undoubtedly, you've heard individuals talking about body fat percentages. Body fat percentiles are arrived at by measuring the amount of fat in one's body against one's total body mass. There are currently three methods that are commonly used. The first, *hydrostatic weighing,* sometimes referred to as underwater weighing, is, however, very difficult to execute. I have done it twice, and both times received an inaccurate reading because I was unable to expel all of the air out of my lungs. Air left in the lungs registers as body fat. You practically have to drown to get an accurate reading. Ironically, this actually is the most reliable technique, but is so difficult for most individuals to perform that its value in the marketplace is limited. For researchers, however, it is easy to implement since they mainly use dissected cadavers, where obviously the issue of air retention in the lungs does not apply.

In addition to the prospect of drowning, some people just do not like placing their head underwater or getting their hair wet. For these individuals this technique should not be considered.

A second technique to measure body fat is termed *bio impedance*. It is performed a couple of ways. An individual steps on a scale and a weak electrical current runs from one foot through the individual's leg and down to the other foot. The slower the current, the more fat the individual possesses. This occurs because fat blocks or impedes the signal. Conversely, the signal travels rapidly through muscle because muscle contains more water than fat, and water conducts electricity. A somewhat more sophisticated bio impedance analysis also exists. It follows a similar but more elaborate protocol. In this technique, the subject reclines and the tester applies four electrodes to the skin. Again, an electrical current is emitted, and as with the body fat scale, the greater the electrical conductance, the less the impedance that is associated with lean body mass, while a lesser electrical conductance suggests impedance of the electric current and is related to a higher body fat mass. A benefit of both of these is that they require little skill on the part of the administrator.

The problem with bio impedance is that you must be in perfect water balance. This rarely occurs, especially when you consider how many individuals are severely dehydrated, or what they ate the previous day, if it contained a good deal of sodium, or if they flew the day before (cabin pressure is extremely dehydrating); or for the female population, at which point they are in their monthly menstrual cycle. Subsequently, it is nearly impossible to get an accurate reading each time when water balance is not a constant.

Skinfold assessment using *calipers* is the third technique, and the most popular employed for body fat percentage measurement. A technician takes measurements at five to seven locations on the body using calipers to measure the thickness of skin folds in millimeters. When the skinfold measurements are properly taken from a variety of body locations, a higher value indicates a greater amount of fat stored beneath the skin and therefore lower body density, and vice versa. The readings are then applied to an appropriate formula to calculate body fat and fat-free mass. To ensure accuracy, the same technician and the same caliper must be used each time the measurement is conducted. Also, note that the accuracy of this reading additionally depends upon the skill of the technician.

Consequently, I have not included body fat measurement as a gauge because it is so fraught with error, both from a human and mechanical standpoint. I definitely rule out underwater weighing and bio impedance. However, if with absolute certainty you can have a fitness professional, friend, or some other individual with experience with skinfold calipers take the measurements, then go ahead. Just don't get hung up on the readings. Use it as an additional gauge. Do the measurement every month, or every other month. But keep in mind, your body measurements by tape measure will clearly reflect your loss of body fat.

STRATEGIC ACTION PLAN

At the start of this chapter we talked about long-term investors and our respect for them and their approach. Just like Warren Buffett's investment strategy, you are embarking upon a long-term weight-loss plan and establishing realistic, attainable "profit" goals. You will revisit the numbers, and through the numbers determine the rate at which you want to lose weight. Examine your present life and make realistic projections of the time, money, and energy it takes to be in the weight-loss business. Then obtain the data, by weighing yourself, being measured, and trying on clothes, thereby establishing a benchmark to gauge your progress. You must be in this for the long haul. This is not a one-day, one-week, one-month, or even a one-year project. This is for life. Your life. Your choice.

Remember, you were patient putting it on, be patient taking it off.

The Business Plan for the Body

Success

IT'S STARTING TO WORK

9 *Taking It On the Road; Keeping It Going*

One of my longest standing clients in Chicago socializes with many of my other clients. She always talks about going to dinner parties or charity events and having my voice in the back of her head. She stands at an hors d'oeuvres buffet and hears me say: "That's death wrapped in phyllo. That will go directly to your thighs. That could shorten your life by a couple of years. That's candle wax in your bloodstream." She always tells me that I ruin everything. Well, my goal is not to ruin everything, but I do want to be a "voice in her head" and I want to keep her from sabotaging her success. I want her to be smart. I want her to be informed. Because of her newfound knowledge, she won't nibble on all the high-caloric foods at the party, but she will love the feeling in the morning when she looks at herself in the mirror or steps on her scale.

Change is inevitable. It occurs in the financial markets, the political world, the fashion world, the weather, and within individuals. It simply cannot be ignored, but it can be managed. You are on plan and clearly on your way to being a smashing success in the weight-loss business. As you continue with your plan, two issues that relate to change need to be addressed. How do you stay successful in the weight-loss business, reach your ultimate goal and continue in business? And how are you

> **"Even if you're on the right track, you'll get run over if you just sit there."**
>
> **WILL ROGERS**

going to manage to stay on plan during a business lunch, a family weekend, a crunch week at the office, or numerous other obstacles and temptations that might sabotage your weight-loss goal? Let's examine these issues individually.

We are in agreement, you are in the weight-loss business. Your goal is to be a success in this venture. Do most companies go into business hoping to go out of business? I would hope not. Have you ever heard a company spokesman proclaim, "Our dream is to go Chapter Eleven"? Are you going into the weight-loss business hoping to go belly up? We know you're not because you went public with your weight-loss intent. But consider past experience. I bet you have lost weight in the past. I also bet you have gained all if not more of it back. What keeps happening? Why can't you keep the weight off? From previous chapters, we know that weight loss is a function of the equation, calories in minus calories out. Previously, you went on a diet, lost some weight, then curtailed the diet and resumed your old eating habits. Consequently, you gained back all if not more of the weight you had lost. Why? On the diet, you were creating a caloric deficit. Your calories in were less than your calories out. You lost weight. But we also know from previous chapters that there are two reasons why your metabolism will slow down when you restrict calories. One, as we have established—when you restrict calories, the body slows down as a defense mechanism to keep you alive. Therefore, your basal metabolic rate declines. Two, unless you were simultaneously doing strength and resistance training in addition to dieting, you lost body fat *and* some lean muscle tissue. A loss of lean muscle tissue translates into a slower metabolism. Therefore, you got hit with a double diminishment to your metabolism.

CHANGE CAN
BE MANAGED
SUCCESSFULLY

So now, after your weight loss, you are burning fewer calories each day at rest. You have a slower metabolism. You resume your old eating habits, which we know contributed to a higher body weight and a greater caloric consumption. Therefore, as you return to your previous eating habits, you are creating a larger caloric *surplus* than before. More "energy" is coming in and less is going out. You are gaining weight faster than ever. You are out of the weight-loss business and back into the weight-gain business with a vengeance.

The Business Plan for the Body

I can't tell you how many clients my firm has assisted in weight loss for an upcoming special occasion. Whether it be a wedding, reunion, bar mitzvah, or birthday, hundreds of people have lost weight with us, spent a fortune in time, money, and effort, only to go off plan after the event and gain the weight back in no time. I know women who have bought exorbitantly expensive outfits for these events and have worn them only on that day, because they never go back down to "event" weight and size. It may take them six solid months or more to lose the twenty-five pounds, and only six weeks to gain it all back. They successfully entered the weight-loss business and then proceeded to go out of business. They didn't know how to continue their success and modify their plan. They couldn't manage change.

DON'T LOSE WEIGHT FOR AN EVENT, LOSE WEIGHT FOR LIFE

Think about the stock of companies in the past that have followed a similar pattern. Let's use Sears, Roebuck as an example. Since I live in Chicago, I closely follow Sears stock. When Arthur Martinez, the former CEO, first arrived on the scene, he instituted significant changes at Sears. He spun off peripheral businesses, such as Allstate Insurance and Dean Witter Financial Services, and proceeded to streamline the core business, which is retail. The management team did a terrific job, and the increased share price reflected such. For a while this formula seemed to be working. Then, the once successful management team began to err. Competition was aggressive and the market environment was changing at both ends of the retail continuum, discount and department store. Sears was caught in the middle, and unfortunately lost many of its core customers to either discounters such as Wal-Mart and Target or to high-end department store retailers. Basically, Sears did not adapt to the changing retail environment. It held on to a formula that for a while had proven successful. The fallout was that Martinez lost his job, though he claims he wanted to retire, and the share price of Sears declined sharply. Had Martinez and Sears management been more savvy of the competition and the rapidly changing market climate, and adjusted their business plan accordingly, this situation would not have happened to the extent that it did. Let me repeat: The management team, led by Martinez, had created a formula for success that worked for a period of time. Unfortunately, the market environment changed but their strategy did not.

Consider some of the other reasons why companies stumble. Say a company is immensely profitable because it aggressively markets and sells to produce strong revenues, meticulously examines expenses to get the best prices, and never takes its eye off the bottom line. What if the CEO, because of bonus and stock options, suddenly becomes a multimillionaire or even a billionaire. He or she may relax, not work as hard, not drive the staff as before, build bigger, more lavish offices, buy a corporate jet, start entertaining more expensively, and cease doing all the things that produced positive results in the past. What happens? You know. I don't have to spell it out for you. You can never take your eye off the bottom line—no pun intended. Both of the previous examples apply as well to the weight-loss business. Just because you are presently experiencing a degree of success does not mean that you can relax with your plan. You must stay focused.

WHEN YOUR ENVIRONMENT CHANGES, YOUR STRATEGY MUST AS WELL

It's important to be very clear on this point. Once you begin the weight-loss business, you are in this business for life. I will again use myself as an illustration. In the previous chapter, we learned that we constantly gauge our success by getting on the scale, taking measurements, and by trying on clothes. I said that when I get on the scale and see that my weight has creeped up, I immediately go on strict plan. That way I never have more than a few pounds to lose. Being on plan means weighing yourself once a week. If you stop weighing yourself, I guarantee your weight will start to creep up. You will be discouraged and disappointed in yourself and ultimately quit your program altogether. We tend to avoid that which is unpleasant. Does this sound like a familiar pattern? The weight-loss business, like all businesses, requires discipline.

Keep in mind, there is no such thing as weight maintenance. Weight maintenance assumes you don't fluctuate in weight. That is impossible. An individual's weight fluctuates all the time; though the fluctuations are not huge, they do occur. Therefore, you are constantly in the weight-loss business because numerous factors can cause you to gain a little weight. In addition, we also know that as we age, our metabolism slows because our body tends to lose lean muscle tissue, which we counteract through strength and resistance training. Our metabolism also slows as a function of the aging process. What will

The Business Plan for the Body

keep you in the weight-loss business is the concept I call *progression*. I have alluded to this term at several points in the book. Allow me now to explain its important contribution to *The Business Plan for the Body*.

Most people fail in the weight-loss business because they do not understand the concept of progression, which is essential to any weight-loss plan and needs to be applied to both components, eating and exercise. Reviewing the facts: The body is very intelligent. We have established that when restricting calories on a daily basis the body slows down metabolically in order to keep you alive. So, if you establish one weight-loss plan and expect your body to continually respond to that one program, you are underestimating your body's intelligence and undermining the concept of being "on plan."

We established in Chapter 2, Fallacy 6, that the body never plateaus, but that weight-loss programs can. I introduced you to the phrase, "confusion facilitates change." We know that when we apply new stimuli to the body it will be forced to adapt and change. If we stay with the same program, ultimately the body will plateau. Remember the example of the woman who lived in my former condominium building and her walking program? Her body hadn't plateaued, her weight-loss program had.

As previously stated, progression needs to be applied to both variables in your metabolic equation, the calories in and the calories out. You established realistic weight-loss goals by working the metabolic equation. You know that to lose weight, you need to create a caloric deficit. If you are continuing to lose weight and meeting your weight-loss projections, then you are appropriately manipulating the equation. But what if your weight loss slows down and the scale stops its downward trend? Then it's time to revisit the Harris-Benedict Basal Metabolic Rate Equation.

Go back to page 63. When was the last time you plugged in your current weight, age, and activity level? My guess is that you haven't done this since you began your plan, so now it's necessary to input the new numbers, taking into consideration your age, if you are older; your weight, which should be lower; and your activity level, which should be higher. For purposes of illustration, let's use a five-foot, ten-inch, 225-pound, fifty-year-old male. For this individual, the original equation was:

65 + (6.22 × weight [lbs.]) + (12.7 × height [inches])
− (6.8 × age) = Basal Metabolic Rate (BMR)
or
65 + (6.22 × 225) + (12.7 × 70) − (6.8 × 50) =
65 + 1399.50 + 889 − 340 = 2,013.50 BMR Calories

Remember, resting metabolic rate refers to the number of calories one's body requires to perform basic vital bodily functions such as breathing, digestion, and the like. Resting metabolic rate also assumes you never got out of bed, but stay awake approximately sixteen hours a day. After six months on *The Business Plan for the Body,* our subject now weighs 185 pounds. His equation now would be as follows:

65 + (6.22 × 185) + (12.7 × 70) − (6.8 × 50)
= New Resting Metabolism
65 + 1150.70 + 889 − 340 = 1,764.70 BMR Calories

After six months the calories burned through his new resting metabolic rate have decreased. But wait, now we need to apply a new activity multiplier since he has begun an exercise program. Remember the following chart:

ACTIVITY MULTIPLIER

Sedentary	1.15 multiplier
Light Activity (normal, everyday activities)	1.3 multiplier
Moderately Active (exercise 3 to 4 times a week)	1.4 multiplier
Very Active (exercise more than 4 times a week)	1.6 multiplier
Extremely Active (exercise 6 to 7 times a week)	1.8 multiplier

Using the number produced by the original equation, 2,013.50 calories burned each day, multiplied by a sedentary activity multiplier, 1.15, his original equation was:

2,013.50 × 1.15 = 2,315.53 Total Calories Burned

Now, using the number produced by the revised equation, taking into consideration his weight loss, multiplied by a moderately active multiplier, 1.4, his new equation is:

1,764.70 × 1.4 = 2,470.58 Total Calories Burned

So he now requires 155.05 more calories per day than he did previously to maintain his present weight. But wait, what about the increase in basal metabolic rate that I told you is derived from the increase in lean muscle tissue that occurs through strength and resistance training? Good question. That will definitely occur. Unfortunately, when the Harris-Benedict equation was devised, the researchers were not aware of the significance of strength and resistance training and did not include the applicable numbers in the equation. As I keep repeating, one pound of lean muscle tissue will burn between 35 to 50 calories per pound, per day. So, if you have put on five pounds of lean muscle tissue through strength and resistance training, you will burn *an additional 175 to 250 calories each day.* This will make a significant difference and is one of the keys to success in the weight-loss business. As you progress in your strength and resistance program, you are building lean muscle tissue and subsequently increasing your basal metabolic rate.

Do you see why dieting without strength and resistance exercise does not work? Do you also see why dieting with only cardiovascular exercise does not work? Given these two scenarios, it would be necessary for you to continue to eat less and less in order to continue to lose weight or do more and more cardiovascular exercise. No one I know can do that nor should they attempt to. That is why strength and resistance exercise is an essential component in the weight-loss business. It is not an option. Only through strength and resistance exercise do you get the benefit of increased daily caloric burning twenty-four hours a day. That is the key to success. Remember our discussion in Chapter 2, which stated that any program that does not promote exercise will ultimately fail. It is almost certain failure to attempt a weight-loss program and keep the weight off without incorporating strength and resistance exercise. That weight-loss program might lead you to improved health, but it will not put you in or keep you in the weight-loss business.

DO THE MATH, LEAN MUSCLE TISSUE BURNS 35 TO 50 CALORIES PER POUND, PER DAY

Also, keep in mind that the previous illustration described program progression as it relates to a male. It is a very different picture for women. First, men are generally bigger than women, so simply as a function of size, they need more calories to fuel their bodies on a daily basis. Second, men have more muscle than women, and we established early on that muscle is the most metabolically active tissue. Third, men and women have a different body composition and possess a different amount of essential body fat. Stay with me a moment on this point.

Men have 3 percent essential body fat and women have 12 percent essential body fat. The biggest reason for this disparity is a female's reproductive system. These organs require body fat to function. This is the reason why women who suffer an eating disorder or who overexercise will frequently cease their monthly menstruation cycle until their body fat returns to the minimum amount required for normal functioning. My point: Even if a man and woman were the same height, weight, and age, the woman would possess more body fat and less muscle than the man.

Consequently, creating a caloric deficit for a woman is somewhat more difficult than for a man. In order to be able to create that caloric deficit, exercise assumes an even greater role in one's weight-loss program. Review the activity multipliers. At a certain point women should strive for four exercise sessions a week to move to the next multiplier. There is a limit as to how many calories you can delete from your eating allocation on a daily basis. It would not be healthy nor is it my recommendation. What you should do is make the time to exercise four times a week, and as we established in Chapter 7, be certain to incorporate lots and lots of strength and resistance training into your program. In the beginning a woman should complete two to three exercise sessions a week, but if her weight starts to plateau, she should strive to achieve an additional hour of strength and resistance training each week.

Also, remember what occurs to women during and after menopause. They begin to lose a full pound of muscle each year. Therefore, only progressive strength and resistance training can halt this lean muscle tissue loss and even build new tissue.

I know this can appear discouraging. You must be thinking, "I do all this work, count my calories, exercise, and put all the time and energy into establishing and implementing my plan, and now you tell me I have to do more!" Well, as I said in my introduction, you may not like some aspects of the plan. I would rather be open and honest with you than trick you into trusting me and then have your plan not produce results.

Yes, as you continue in the weight-loss business you will have to work harder. The original pounds, probably the same pounds you have gained and lost dozens if not hundreds of times, are the easy pounds. The hard work comes later, down the road, when it is not as easy to create a caloric deficit because your body weight is lower. Remember when I said early on: For people who are overweight and overeating, losing the initial five to ten pounds is easy. As you proceed with the plan, the body does put up somewhat of a fight.

Recall when you were in the weight-gain business. You were working harder and harder to put weight on. Though it may not have seemed that difficult to you, it was occurring. Think about it. Ironically, you were participating in progression. You were consuming more and more calories and therefore progressing your caloric intake and increasing your body weight. Had you ceased that progression, you would have maintained your weight. This is especially true of people who put on a great deal of weight in a relatively short period of time.

Let me elaborate. I established earlier that the human body does not want to be overweight. Only by overeating and under-exercising can the body increase in weight. But when you go on a restricted calorie diet, the body slows down in order to keep you alive. It is as if the body does not know that you are carrying so much additional "energy" or fat. So in the weight-loss business, the body will fight you, but you can fight back. How? You guessed it: strength and resistance exercises.

For example, let's say that you successfully lost weight on plan, but now the pounds aren't coming off as quickly or you reached a plateau. What can you do? First, review your present eating program. In other words, your calories in. Apply pro-gression to your eating plan (and by progression, I don't mean eating more, I mean eating less). Where can you delete a few additional calories? Should you increase your fruit and veg-etable consumption? Are you taking too many liberties with your eating? Frequently, I see individuals start their weight-loss program and follow it to the letter. After a while they start to cheat a little, not count their calories as diligently, splurge much too often. Don't follow that pattern. Be truthful. If you were ini-tially keeping the food diary and became sloppy with your recording, this is the time to reinstate the diary and obtain "the data." Are you eating out too frequently? Restaurant food is generally higher in calories than what you are eating at home and less within your control. If you socialize often, start entertaining at home more or specifically at restaurants where they are amenable to your specific needs. That way, you are in control. Also consider your water consumption. Make sure you are drinking as much as possible throughout the day. Water consumption will always make a difference in weight loss and in your appearance.

FIND WAYS TO SHAVE A FEW ADDITIONAL CALORIES

Now assess your exercise allocation. Are you getting as many workouts in as possible? Are you doing 25 percent cardiovascular exercise and 75 percent strength and resistance training? And most important, are you progressing your program?

Remember Your Exercise Allocation
25% Cardiovascular and 75% Strength and Resistance Training

Keep in mind, progression is the essential component to a successful strength and resistance program in the weight-loss business. Begin with the basics. When you first did the lat pulldown exercise pictured on page 138, your back and bicep muscles were challenged. You struggled to perform perhaps fifteen repetitions with the green Xertube band. As the days or weeks pass and you are consistently exercising, a time will come when it becomes easy for you to perform fifteen repetitions of the lat pulldown with this tube. That's the time to progress your strength and resistance program. You can accomplish progression through any or all of the following methods.

METHODS OF PROGRESSION

INCREASE THE WEIGHT OR THE TENSION OF THE BAND

The simplest way to progress your strength and resistance program is to increase your training poundage or band tension. Always increase by the smallest increment. With free weights that would translate into going from three pounds to five to eight to ten, etc. The same applies to a weight machine, which

The Business Plan for the Body

usually increases in five-pound increments, though many new machines may go up by a 2.5-pound increment. With the Spri Xertubes this would translate into going to the higher tension band, advancing from yellow to green, red, blue, then ultimately black. You can also increase the tension of the band by stepping farther away from the band's point of attachment. Keep in mind, progression does not mean that you must perform all repetitions with the higher weight and/or tension. Using a bicep curl as an example, you may have been performing fifteen repetitions with eight-pound weights. To progress to the ten-pound weights, you may be able to perform some of the repetitions with the higher weight, say ten repetitions, then drop down to the eight-pound weights to complete the final five repetitions of the set. This is important to remember. Always start with the heavier weight, and as you begin to fatigue and almost fail, drop to the lower weight or tension or just stop at failure. Don't begin with a light weight and plan during the set to increase to a heavier one when your muscle is beginning to fatigue.

PROGRESS REALISTICALLY

Similar to unrealistic weight-loss expectations, don't place undue pressure on your body to immediately be able to jump up in weight and/or band tension. Be aware of the percentage increase. When you go from eight- to ten-pound weights, you are actually increasing your training poundage by 25 percent. That is a substantial increase. So, simultaneously, keep the percentages in mind as you increase the actual weight.

Just a side note. Most free weights are similar, but all machines are not created equal. If you are using brand-name strength and resistance equipment, such as Cybex or Life Fitness, the tension on the same machine in one setting may be slightly different on another because of the tension of the cable. Or you may be doing fifty pounds for an exercise on one brand of equipment, but barely able to do forty pounds on another brand. Just be smart. Adjust the weight accordingly. Don't overdo it, which frequently leads to injury. Think.

INCREASE THE REPETITIONS

With most exercises, I feel that a maximum of fifteen repetitions should be performed. After fifteen repetitions your joints may be at risk of injury, so that's why I say to stop there. But if you are not yet at fifteen repetitions, then progress until you get there. When you reach fifteen, you will have to adjust one of the other variables. Ideally, I want you to perform between twelve and fifteen repetitions of most exercises.

For your information, many exercise classes encourage their participants to perform way too many repetitions. I should know, as years ago I used to teach dozens of classes a week. Currently, there is a class called "body pump" that advocates over a hundred repetitions of many exercises. Attending such classes is an easy route to an injury because the human body's joints were not created to perform these excessive repetitions. I would actually recommend that physical therapists and orthopedic surgeons stand outside these classes and pass out their business cards. I know I am sounding a bit extreme, but please, don't believe that you are in the weight-loss business by frequently attending these classes. You're not. Be smart and avoid injury.

BEWARE OF EXERCISE CLASSES

Exercise classes, in general, are not the quickest way to weight loss. Sure, they are fun. Every now and then I jump into a spin or step class since the music is loud, the energy is contagious, and I need a little mental boost. I do the class because I enjoy it. But by no means do I believe that the class will make me a success in the weight-loss business. I do it for enjoyment, just as someone may play golf, tennis, bowl, or swim leisurely. Exercise classes simply cannot effectively incorporate progression and lean muscle tissue building. They also cannot be custom-designed to your specific needs, since the nature of a class is to appeal to a wide variety of members.

INCREASE THE NUMBER OF SETS

As we established in Chapter 7, you should begin with a one-set protocol. But as you progress you may feel that a second set is justified. You can do the second set (also with up to fifteen repetitions) right after the first, or you can circuit-train, as I do, and do one set of all your exercises and then repeat. I enjoy circuit training. It involves doing exercise after exercise with limited time in between. You move. Though I have only allocated 25 percent of your exercise to straight cardiovascular exercise, you are receiving additional cardio by circuit training, since your heart rate will stay elevated throughout your strength and resistance program. So, as you circuit train, you get the benefits of increasing your lean muscle tissue plus some additional caloric burning through cardiovascular exercise. Circuit training is a challenging way to exercise, both to your mind and body, and the session passes quickly. There is nothing better to me than a workout when the time flies by. Like most individuals, I really don't like exercise, but I *love* the results, both in the way I look and feel.

REDUCE THE SPEED

This is the most often neglected element of progression. You should employ a two-count positive motion followed by a two-count negative. In other words, for a bicep curl, that would translate to two counts as you slowly lift the weight up and two counts as you slowly lower the weight back down to your side. In technical terms the lifting phase is the *concentric* motion and the lowering phase is the *eccentric* phase. To incorporate additional progression to an exercise, you may choose to go to a three-, four-, or five-count speed. Numerous studies believe that the most effective way to take all the momentum out of an exercise and challenge a muscle in the safest possible manner is to do ten-count repetitions, both positive and negative. Now, these are very hard. I don't recommend this protocol for a beginner. But as you continue with your plan, this may be a viable option. Don't neglect decreasing the speed of each repetition. It also is one of the *safest* ways to progress your plan.

SPEED IS AN OVERLOOKED VARIABLE TO ACHIEVE PROGRESSION

CHANGE THE ANGLE

An additional way to progress your plan is to change the angle of the exercise. Using the squat as an example, as illustrated on page 145, my plan included a squat with toes forward and in alignment with your knees. A simple way to progress this exercise is to turn the toes out. All of a sudden you are challenging your muscles at a different angle and placing additional emphasis on the inner thigh, which frequently is an area many females wish to improve. This exercise would resemble a classic plié from ballet class. Same movement, weight, repetitions, sets, speed, and stability, but different stimulation and recruitment of muscle fiber. Another example is the lat pulldown.

What would happen if you turned your palms over and had them face up rather than down? All of a sudden a new angle is created that challenges the muscle further. See the point? Slight changes are all you need. These are not new exercises, just the same exercise with a slight twist. That change in angle confuses the muscle further.

A word of caution regarding changing the angle of exercises. This concept does become a bit tricky and technical. If you are a beginner, I would employ other avenues of progression. You can increase the intensity, the reps, the sets, or the speed before changing the angle of the exercise. I recommend that you not alter the angle until you can successfully perform the exercises and isolate the muscle groups for twelve weeks.

ADD INSTABILITY

As you saw from Chapter 7, I included a Resist-a-ball as part of your equipment. A fit ball is a terrific way to incorporate instability into an exercise. To illustrate, let's use the dumbbell bench-chest press. Normally, when performing this exercise, you lie down on a stationary bench, place the two dumbbells in each hand, and slowly press the weights up over your head. You are stimulating the chest, or pectoral muscles, as the primary mover, and the back of the arms, the triceps, as the secondary mover. Consider what would happen if you performed this exercise on a fit ball in place of a stationary bench. Immediately your abdominals and lower back muscles are called into play in order to maintain proper position on the ball. In addition, your gluteus maximus (your rear end) needs to assist your body to stay up, as well as the front of your legs, the quadriceps, and the back of the legs, the hamstrings. Then as you start to press the weights up, lying on this unstable surface requires you to use even more of the pectoral and tricep muscles, as you must both lift the weights *and* control the movement on that unstable surface. You will recruit additional muscle fiber to complete the motion. Therefore, you will stimulate the muscle more than you would on a stable surface where the issue of balance is not a factor. This is a perfect way to progress a program and really challenge your muscles. An added plus is that I find the ball is actually more comfortable on my back when I perform certain exercises.

INSTABILITY RECRUITS ADDITIONAL MUSCLE FIBER, WHICH BUILDS LEAN MUSCLE TISSUE

The Business Plan for the Body

Another exercise that easily lends itself to the incorporation of instability is the lunge. To create that instability, my fitness training firm often uses a half piece of foam when performing lunges. Basically, think of a cylinder of foam cut in half. There is a flat side and a rounded side. By placing either the front or back foot on the flat side of the half foam, facing up with the rounded side facing down, you generate instability in the lunge. Your muscles have to work much harder to stabilize as you slowly move up and down. Once again, this further challenges the muscles and stimulates additional muscle fiber.

CHANGE EQUIPMENT

If you regularly work out in a health club, exercise room, park district, or other setting, your program most likely will be executed on weight machines and the same rules of progression apply. You can easily progress your plan by increasing the weight by the smallest increment, increasing your repetitions up to fifteen, doing additional sets of the same exercise, slowing down the speed, or changing the angle. The only progression that may not be as easy to incorporate is the instability factor, because most machines are fixed and should only be used in the manner in which they were designed. But a large facility, loaded with numerous weight training machines, possesses a very significant progression component—you can perform the same movements on a different brand of weight machine. As an example for those of you familiar **INTELLIGENTLY** with weight machines, a seated hamstring curl is **USE A VARIETY** quite different from a prone (or on your stomach) **OF EQUIPMENT** hamstring curl. Both machines isolate the hamstring muscle, but the resistance is coming from the two very distinct angles and movements. So if you regularly work out in an exercise facility, use the equipment, then challenge yourself to stimulate the same muscle groups using completely different equipment. Or you could simply move from machines to free weights, which, as earlier discussed, challenge the user to both stabilize the weight and place resistance against a muscle.

BUILD AND EXECUTE A PERIODIZATION PROGRAM

A what? Periodization? Okay, don't be intimidated by the terminology. Periodization is a very intelligent, basic way to incorporate progression into your exercise program. Here is how it works: Select a group of exercises designed for the body parts you wish to stimulate. Then, for the next eight weeks, perform the same exercises each week. Throughout the eight weeks attempt to increase the weight, the reps, and the number of sets. The goal of this program is to ultimately lift as much weight and subsequently build as much muscle as possible. The Strategic Exercise Plan I gave you in Chapter 7 is basically your first periodization program. So, over the next eight weeks, continue with this plan and increase the weight once you can perform fifteen repetitions with ease. You will be amazed how your strength increases, and it is highly motivating to experience this progression. After eight weeks stop that program and build another. You can use all the concepts I outlined for you in Chapter 7, just build a completely new program. Either do completely different exercises that specifically target the muscles you need to build, or change the current exercises by adjusting the angles either through the point of tension or the hand grip or by adding instability where you can, and presto, you have a new periodization program. I strongly urge you to do a periodization. This style of training produces great results and makes it very easy to document your progress on the plan. Once the plan is devised, all you have to do is execute and progress it. Simple. As I keep saying, a strength and resistance program is not difficult to implement once you learn the few variables that need to be addressed to derive the maximum benefits from strength and resistance training.

PERIODIZATION
IS A BASIC WAY
TO ASSURE
PROGRESSION

Going on a periodization is a choice. Personally, I devise an eight-week periodization with my trainer, complete it, then go off periodization for a few weeks before developing a new one. Mind you, I go off periodization, not off strength and resistance training. I like the balance because I find it both mentally and physically challenging to mix things, on periodization and off. The choice is yours. Just remember to always document the exercise, the weight, the repetitions, the sets, the speed, and the angle, to apply effective progression either on or off periodization.

Don't allow this discussion of periodization to confuse you. If you are a beginner, just follow the Strategic Exercise Plan for

The Business Plan for the Body

the first eight weeks and then regroup. For intermediate to advanced exercisers, you probably already understand this concept.

USE SCHEDULING TO YOUR ADVANTAGE

In the scheduling section of Chapter 7, I mentioned that when forced to schedule exercise sessions on back-to-back days your plan would have to be modified. That is accomplished by doing the following: If, because of scheduling, you plan to exercise on both Saturday and Sunday or other consecutive days, split your workout by either doing the first half of your program on Saturday and the second half on Sunday, or you can do all the lower body exercises on Saturday and the upper body on Sunday. Keep in mind, you should do twice as many exercises for those body parts since you are only doing half the program. I want you to get the same amount of exercise time in each day. This is actually a good solution since you will force these muscles to work harder than usual because you'll be working them twice as long. It should not be an issue when you have to work out on back-to-back days, and should not deter you from staying on plan. As I said, many busy people, especially those who travel a great deal during the week, do back-to-back weekend workouts. That keeps them in the weight-loss business. You easily can do the same.

CARDIOVASCULAR EXERCISE CAN ALSO BENEFIT FROM PROGRESSION

Thus, the entire concept of progression is simple. You must keep challenging your muscles. This will lead to an increase in your lean muscle tissue, and, yes, for almost the last time, an increase in your basal metabolic rate, which creates increased caloric burning twenty-four hours a day. You may be asking, "But what about cardiovascular exercise? Do I have to progress that as well?" Absolutely.

PROGRESSING YOUR CARDIOVASCULAR PROGRAM

During my discussion of cardiovascular exercise, I explained your body's oxygen transportation system. As you perform an exercise, say walking, your large muscles in the lower body require oxygen to perform the activity. The oxygen is transported by blood, and the blood is pumped by the heart. Presto, your heart rate is elevated. But what happens over time? The same adaptation that takes place through strength and resistance training. Once the body is efficient at supplying oxygen to the working muscles, it does not have to work as hard and subsequently will burn fewer calories. You and I know you want to burn more calories. Therefore, you must also progress your cardiovascular exercise. Here are your options:

INCREASE YOUR SPEED

By increasing the speed, whether it be walking outside or on a treadmill, or the revolutions per minute on a bike, StairMaster, or elliptical trainer, you increase the intensity of the exercise. I urged you to purchase a heart rate monitor. This device will give you the information you require to adjust your speed accordingly. Or you can always take a manual heart rate. When you began your program, you walked at 3.5 miles per hour with your heart rate at 140 beats per minute. Now, moving at the same speed, your heart rate only elevates to 120 beats per minute. You've just witnessed progress. Your body is now more efficient in supplying oxygen to the working muscles. So what is it time to do? Increase the exercise intensity and get your heart rate back up. Why? This will enable you to continue to burn more calories and further challenge your cardiovascular system.

INCREASE THE INTENSITY

By increasing the intensity, whether by elevating the incline on a treadmill, walking outside in a hilly area, or increasing the tension on a bike, StairMaster, or elliptical trainer, you increase the load on the muscles and subsequently the need for more oxygen to be supplied to the working muscles. This is not the same as increasing the speed at which you perform the exercise. This is the intensity. Think of biking up a hill. You are not going faster, but you are working harder because of the incline. Once again, a heart rate monitor will immediately indicate when there is an increase in intensity and respond accordingly. Previously, I urged you to increase the speed to apply progression. But after a while it does not make sense to attempt to go faster. It makes much better sense to increase the intensity, and will also be easier on your joints over time.

The Business Plan for the Body

CROSS-TRAIN

Most people do not understand the concept of cross-training. Basically, it means performing a variety of physical activities. If you walk, then start biking; if you bike, then climb stairs; if you use an elliptical trainer, then swim. Every time you change the activity, you challenge your muscles a different way and thus cross-train. Play singles tennis, which years ago was classified as an aerobic activity, get yourself in a rowboat and move those oars, anything that is different from what you generally do for your cardiovascular exercise. Cross-training also preserves your joints, since repetitive motions, such as constant running or cycling, can wear out your joints over time. I also urge people when traveling or at a different exercise facility to try out some of the equipment they don't regularly use in their home, office, or exercise facility. Seize the opportunity to cross-train.

PARTICIPATION IN A VARIETY OF ACTIVITIES CAN PRESERVE YOUR JOINTS

CAUTION
Please avoid rowing machines. They can be hazardous to your lower back. The only exception would be the Concept II Rowing Machine, which truly resembles a rowing motion.

As previously mentioned, in addition to the cardiovascular benefits, cross-training also saves your joints from overuse injuries. Since you are working your muscles from different angles and with varying tension, you will keep your muscles and joints in balance and prevent injury over time.

INSTABILITY

Just as instability applies progression in a strength and resistance program, it does much the same for cardiovascular exercise. Think about it. Go for a walk on a hard surface, then hit the soft sand and continue at the same pace. Instantly your heart rate will go up, since you are on an unstable surface and recruiting additional muscles and muscle fiber to perform the activity. A mountain hike provides both hills, for an increase in intensity, and an uneven surface, which further challenges the muscles. The same applies to biking on a gravel path rather than on cement or asphalt. Climb uneven stairs outside or alternate between single stairs or do every other stair, as I did for years with clients at a few monuments in Chicago's Lincoln Park, and once again your body is forced to work harder as it adjusts to stairs of varying heights.

The following are a few misconceptions regarding progressing both a strength and resistance program and a cardiovascular program.

MISCONCEPTIONS REGARDING PROGRESSION

You have to run to burn calories. No, you don't. But why do some people believe running is the only answer? That's simple— intensity. Running is very intense. It places high demand on the heart to pump blood to the working muscles. But can't you work at a high intensity on any piece of cardiovascular equipment? Yes, yes, yes. Running is not the only activity that is high in intensity. Other high-intensity activities include stair stepping, biking, swimming, or just about any cardiovascular exercise that is performed aggressively. Just adjust the variables I previously outlined during any cardiovascular exercise and derive the same intensity as running, with less risk of injury to one's joints.

NO, YOU DON'T HAVE TO RUN TO BURN CALORIES

Frequently, I have people say to me, "I used to run, which really kept my weight down. Now I have bad knees, can't run, so I gave up." Here is my analysis of running. For a certain population, running is fine. These individuals have the alignment and structure that allows the joints to withstand the constant pounding of running. For them, running is appropriate. Unfortunately, very few people possess the alignment that will enable them to repeatedly run without injury.

If I progress my strength and resistance program, I will injure myself. This is absolutely untrue. Just as I described in Chapter 7 when I encouraged you to begin my program, using small increments of progression and listening to your body when something doesn't feel right, you will not get injured. Attempt to progress too rapidly, and you increase your chances of injury. Listen to a friend who does not know what he or she is talking about and is using a strength and resistance program they developed in the 1970s, and once again your chances of sustaining an injury increase.

PAIN IS NOT THE SAME AS SORENESS

The Business Plan for the Body

Note, there is a difference between pain and soreness. When you first begin to exercise, especially strength and resistance exercises, you will most likely experience some muscular soreness lasting for a day or two after the workout. This is common. Your muscles are simply telling you that they have not been challenged in a long time. This soreness will dissipate in a few days. This is normal. Lasting pain (not muscular soreness) that you feel in a muscle or joint is not normal and requires immediate medical attention and should not be ignored.

Throughout this book I have brought up the concept of listening to your body. Frequently, I hear people complain about injuries. I generally ask, "When did you first start to experience pain?" Most of the time the individuals will tell me that their knee, back, neck, or some other body part started to bother them a long time ago. They simply chose to ignore it, hoping it would just go away. Pain is an indication that something is wrong, whether as the result of an accident, alignment problem, or simply overuse. Listen to your body. If you are in pain, even slight pain, that may escalate in the future and possibly curtail your program. Be smart. If something doesn't feel right, stop. If necessary, take a little time off to see if the problem subsides. Don't perform any exercise that simply feels wrong.

Progression is just too hard. This is and is not true. Let's use the example of climbing the corporate ladder. Your first position was basically an entry-level position. Did you have that much job responsibility and related stress? Probably not. As you climbed the ladder, promotion after promotion, did the job get more difficult as you assumed more and more responsibility? Most likely it did. Was the effort worth the gain? I assume all your hard work has paid off in professional satisfaction, financial rewards, and enhanced self-esteem. Would you have been content to stay at your entry-level position? Of course not. Yes, progression is difficult, but the rewards derived are so great that I promise you it will be well worth the results and far outweigh the negatives.

THE ART OF ANTICIPATION
HOW TO STAY ON PLAN IN ANY SITUATION

Now that you have a better feel for progressing your eating and exercise program, let's take a look at the second point I

193

raised at the beginning of this chapter—managing life with all its obstacles and temptations. How do you get through a stressful week at the office, constant travel, a wedding weekend, or many other situations that may divert you from your plan. First of all, you *anticipate*. The following represent a few of the situations and temptations you undoubtedly will encounter, and some suggestions on how to deal with them.

FOOD AT YOUR HOME OR OFFICE

You go to your office. You skipped breakfast, something you should never do. As you're en route, you realize you're starving. You know that each morning, the office sideboard is loaded with huge bagels slathered with cream cheese, muffins, Danish, juice, and numerous other high-caloric items. So on your way to the office, quickly run into a convenience or grocery store and grab a few pieces of fruit, a yogurt, or even a small bag of pretzels. Suddenly, you are back on plan. No problem. No damage done. No need to be tempted by office food. You anticipated and made a conscious decision to stay on plan.

This same situation applies after taking the kids to school. You're hungry. There is nothing at home, so you decide to stop and get coffee. You go to the counter. There, staring you in the eye, is a bounty of muffins, scones, tarts, bagels, and cookies. You're starving. Don't even think about ordering something other than coffee, not even a latte or cappuccino unless it is made with skim milk, and keep your hands away from the free sample. A "sample" can be the tip of the iceberg and lead to a disaster. Close your eyes, grab your coffee, and run.

Here is how I deal with situations like this when I am out and about. For years I fitness-trained seven to eight clients every day, seven days a week. Every day, I packed a bag with low-calorie items, easy things to carry and eat, such as apples, bananas, oranges, small bags of pretzels, and similar foods. This way, between rushing to clients, I never got stuck without food, never experienced hunger pangs, and subsequently was not tempted to detour from my plan. I wasn't tempted to buy a bag of chips or cookies or some other high-caloric food because I was prepared.

It's not so hard. Thinking on your feet, a quick duck into a store, planning your food in advance, and you stay on plan.

Ignore it, pretend that hunger doesn't exist, and your plan comes apart. Why? Because you allowed it. You didn't anticipate. Remember, you *can* be the man or woman with the plan. You just have to make the commitment to yourself.

Just like progression, the entire idea of planning is not difficult. You simply don't allow the situation to take control. You control the situation. According to John Jakicic, Ph.D., of Brown University's Weight Control and Diabetes Research Center, "If you don't have your environment and infrastructure in place, all the willpower in the world won't work."

THE BUSINESS DINNER

If you are stressed and busy at home or the office and have to go to a business dinner that starts with hors d'oeuvres at seven-thirty and you had lunch at noon, anticipate and eat a late afternoon snack: a piece of fruit, a yogurt, an energy bar, or anything else that fills you up so you don't attend the event hungry. If you do arrive famished, you will undoubtedly consume thousands of calories of hors d'oeuvres *before* the dinner because you are starving. Don't do it. Plan ahead.

THE DINNER PARTY

You know the host well and they're aware you've *gone public* with your plan. You phone your host and say, "I hate to be a pest and I'm so thrilled to be invited to your dinner, but can you do me a favor? Is it possible to serve my salad with the dressing on the side, my entrée with the sauce on the side, etc. Please, don't think I am requesting a completely different meal. Just a few adjustments. It would really mean a great deal to me if you helped me out. You know how important this plan is to me." What mentally "healthy" host or hostess would not be happy to oblige? After all, they invited you. Be polite, be sweet, and be clear with your needs. You're not being finicky, so you shouldn't be embarrassed. Most likely, your fellow diners will be interested in your success story.

> DON'T ALLOW THE SITUATION TO TAKE CONTROL . . . *YOU* CONTROL THE SITUATION

If you feel uncomfortable calling your host or this is a business acquaintance, try the following: First, do not go to their home hungry. Plan ahead and have a light snack of baby carrots, a yogurt, some fruit, a plain baked potato, or something else you like that will partially fill you up before you go. When you arrive, skip the hors d'oeuvres, since they are usually loaded with fat and calories, unless they are crudités, and in that case avoid the dip. When the meal comes, pick around it. Try to push dressing and sauce to the side. By all means, skip the mashed potatoes (for a few years, a chic local caterer in Chicago constantly served mashed potatoes that consisted of a pound of butter, a pound of cream, and a pound of potatoes) and other items that you know are loaded with calories and fat. Same with dessert—skip it or just have a few bites. Most people will not notice how much you ate. If someone does make a comment, then politely *go public* for them. Just eat as little as possible and then plan on a light, healthy snack at home. Once again, you just turned a potential disaster into a minor adjustment.

THE BUFFET LINE

You are a guest at a hotel or resort or a holiday brunch. Not a problem. Fill up on the fruit tray, which is always available, vegetables and a salad without the dressing, then include a few of your favorites in portion-controlled sizes. Most buffets have sliced white meat turkey or chicken, which we know keeps you right on plan, or vegetable omelettes made to order, which can be done with egg whites or any other egg substitute and prepared in nonstick spray. You have just taken a potentially horrible situation and turned it into a winner. What to avoid? Definitely all high-calorie carbohydrates such as muffins, pastries, and croissants, the greasy breakfast meats such as sausage, ham, bacon, and Canadian bacon. You should also avoid the high-mayonnaise items such as egg, tuna, or chicken salad.

If available, look for a smaller, salad-size plate to begin the buffet. If you start with an entrée-size plate, odds are you will fill it up. So start smaller, eat slowly, don't let others at the table tempt you with all their high-fat choices, and enjoy.

BIG EVENTS

What about an out-of-town wedding, a family reunion, the holidays? First of all, start each day with fruit and an egg white omelette in nonstick spray. If you have to attend a planned meal, ask the waiter if a fruit plate is available in lieu of the prearranged meal or if your salad can have dressing on the side. I frequently do this when I go to weddings, benefits, or other similar functions. I ask my waiter, politely, if he or she could bring me an alternative meal or just leave the sauce and dressing off the dinner. It's easy. Be assertive. Don't get your food and say, "Gee, I guess I have to eat the Caesar salad with dressing and the chicken in cream sauce because that's all they're serving." Wrong. With a slight adjustment, you greatly reduce the amount of calories you consume. Be proactive. Control your environment and your caloric allocation, don't let it control you. Don't be a victim. Be a winner. Skip the wedding cake or dessert, or once again have a few bites. Suddenly, the disaster event becomes a no brainer. You have the routine. You have a plan and thus you have the power.

I touched upon this concept earlier and want to revisit it. As you become a success in the weight-loss business, people will take you seriously. When you ask a host or hostess to make slight adjustments, they, too, will learn about your plan. They will respect you. You are becoming a smashing success. When you are attending a charity benefit or restaurant and your "light" dinner arrives, others at the table will try to order the same. This happens to me all the time. Half the people at the table say, "Hey, where did you get that?" I simply tell them, "I asked."

AIRLINE FOOD

My firm had a client a few years back who was in the business of supplying airline food. Guess what, he never ate it. The standard airline food is a fat, sodium, and caloric nightmare. What you can do is order a special meal in advance. When booking your flight, request a fruit plate or low-calorie meal. Don't order the low-sodium, low-cholesterol, or vegetarian meal and expect it to be low-calorie. It isn't. A fruit plate may be your best bet. Just plan in advance, or get on the plane after a meal and simply decline what is served. Or buy a healthy meal at the airport or en route and skip the plane food. The choice is yours.

RESERVE THE FLIGHT *AND* THE FOOD

THE KIDS

I am a parent. I spend a great deal of time with other parents, especially as my current weekend social life revolves around children's birthday parties. There is junk food everywhere: pizza, chips, fries, cupcakes, brownies, and other assorted caloric disasters. I watch my fellow parents eating this food constantly, whether they take a plate for themselves or, more likely, eat off their child's plate. Stop it. You aren't even thinking as you eat and you're definitely not allocating your calories as you finish off all these foods.

SET A GREAT EXAMPLE FOR THE KIDS

This food is not healthy for you or for your children, and should be eaten sparingly by everyone. In addition to the parties, stop finishing off your kids' food in general. None of them clean their plates, nor should they be encouraged to. (I can't tell you how many men in particular had parents who insisted that they clean their plates. Now, as sixty-year-old successful men, they continue to do so out of guilt and routine.) Wrap the food, put it in the refrigerator, or, while I personally hate to waste food, throw it out. Just don't take it upon yourself to finish every bit that is left over, and in the process destroy your eating allocation and your plan.

Plus, what you eat sets an example for your children. I constantly see overweight parents raising overweight children. Don't even try the genetic argument. Encourage your children to eat a healthy diet, one loaded with fruits and vegetables, and make the burgers, fries, pizza, and the like more the exception than the rule. That way, if you *do* eat from their plate, you will just get an extra serving of fruits or vegetables.

TRIGGER SITUATIONS OR PEOPLE

You know what I am talking about: the parent, sibling, ex-partner or spouse, the reunion, the individuals or situations that historically cause you to go off plan. I have asked you repeatedly to think about your psychological relationship with food. Now you have to be specific. You have to plan. If your "thin" sister is going to be at a holiday dinner, then plan to exercise that day and relieve stress—you should be exercising on holidays anyway, because there generally is nothing to do but eat, drink, sleep, watch television, or some other passive activity—and eat a little something before you arrive at the event. Don't go starving and stressed. That will only lead to a binge, and probably a world-class one. Remember, you went public. You should have no problem being honest about your plan and your strategy to achieve your ultimate

DON'T ALLOW "TRIGGERS" TO BANKRUPT YOUR PLAN

The Business Plan for the Body

goal: weight loss. Early on, when I used Bill Gates and Martha Stewart as examples, I said they not only had a goal, but a strategy to achieve that goal. You can do the same.

If you start to feel stressed at the event, take a deep breath. If you find yourself starting to overeat, excuse yourself from the table, go into another room, and give yourself a pep talk. Respond to your emotion, don't try to push it away with food.

ALCOHOL

A great many social situations include alcohol. In Chapter 6, I noted that wine is 25 calories an ounce and hard liquor is 100 calories an ounce. You have to decide, in both your allocation and in the appropriateness of the event, how much you are going to drink. You also have to decide who is going to drive home. Something I generally do is match two ounces of water for every ounce of wine. That way I don't drink too much and I avoid the dehydrating effect of alcohol when it is broken down by the body. Another idea is to drink spritzers—part wine, part sparkling water—or a light beer. Once again you cut down on the alcohol and the calories but enjoy having a drink that lasts a long time.

Other people I know do best with one vodka, gin, scotch, etc., on the rocks, which they sip all night as they continually add more ice. If this works for you, and your total alcohol allocation is one ounce of hard liquor, great. Keep the portion in control. Just a side note, olives are about 40 calories each and are loaded in fat. So, if you are drinking something that comes with an olive, ask the bartender to hold it. One more idea. Put your water or spritzer in a great glass. I drink sparkling water all the time in a big wineglass. It just makes it more festive to drink out of that glass with a twist of lemon or lime.

DRINK TWO OUNCES OF WATER FOR EVERY OUNCE OF ALCOHOL

And remember, liquid calories do not tip satiation mechanisms in the body. Therefore, even though you are consuming calories when you drink alcohol, the body is not responding and diminishing hunger, as it would if you ate the calories. Plus, alcohol frequently loosens your resolve, which may lead to overeating. So beware.

Just as with strength and resistance training, behavior has components of progression as well. Progression consists of

It's Starting to Work

planning. It consists of anticipation. It consists of intelligence. It requires discipline. This is your choice. You are in control of what goes into your mouth.

STRATEGIC ACTION PLAN

Remember, progression is threefold.

- With regard to food, you need to make sure you stay on top of your allocation. If you become lax, I promise you, your body will once again appear lax. Listen to your body, weigh yourself, try clothing on, take body measurements. If you start to backslide, go back to the food diary and put yourself back on plan.

- You need to keep progressing your strength and resistance program. Once your body stops changing, you know that your program is in need of modification. Keep confusing it. Keep challenging it. Keep forcing your body to build lean muscle tissue. Muscles are big caloric spenders. Use them. Build them.

- Progressing through difficult situations is, more than anything else, about being assertive, confident, and anticipating. Once again, as you become a success, people will listen to you and respect you.

To recap: Change is inevitable. One cannot avoid it, but you can successfully manage and deal with it. You now understand the concept of progression and apply it to all aspects of your plan. You have been provided with suggestions to assist you in dealing with your external environment and the caloric temptations that are out there. I'm sure, as you continue with your plan, you will experience additional situations that require special handling. Just always take a moment to collect your thoughts and proceed intelligently. Think.

I DID IT, I DID IT

10

Now What Do I Do?

After thirteen years in the fitness industry, I believe I have almost seen it all. The successful losers, the not so successful losers, the brief losers, the "event" losers, and the frightened losers. Yes, there are even those who lost weight, became frightened at the prospect of being a slimmer, healthier, attractive person, and immediately regained the weight they lost. So now I ask you: Which loser are you? Funny, this is one of the only events in your life that to be a loser is to be a winner. Are you a happy loser? Are you committed to staying in the weight-loss business? Is this your new plan for life?

Congratulations, you are a success in the weight-loss business. I never doubted your ability to succeed. Only you did. Each and every person has it within their power to change their health, appearance, and body weight. What separates the successes from the failures is the formulation and execution of the plan. So now, every morning, you get out of bed and see the "new" you. How does it feel? I'd guess a little strange at first. I remember as a child not wanting to take my T-shirt off at the pool or beach. I had what was lovingly referred to as a "pot" belly. To this day, when I get invited to a pool party, or I'm going to the beach or hotel pool, my first thought is, "Do I want to wear a bathing suit?" Well yes, I say, but isn't it funny

> **"I did it,
> I did it."**
>
> **OLIVIA KARAS**

that at forty years of age my knee-jerk response is to doubt my appearance, and more important, my self-confidence in a bathing suit. I like my body now. The "pot" is long gone, but the feeling remains. I'm the "Ten-Thousand-Dollar-a-Week Fitness Trainer," yet that feeling was ingrained in me years ago. These are the "tapes" that are hard to erase.

I frequently use that expression, "the tapes." Each of us has an extensive library of internal tapes that are nothing more than our past experiences, memories, and responses. Previously in Chapter 1, I urged you to examine the psychological barriers that may be keeping you from achieving success in the weight-loss business. I believe, both consciously and subconsciously, that many of our present actions are dictated by our past mental tapes. From my experience, very, very few people have non-emotionally related eating and exercise habits. Many clients over the years have conveyed stories of a nagging mother who constantly harped about food, weighed them, and restricted food accordingly. They made body weight a major issue. Or a gym teacher who yelled at a young boy, "You can't run worth s--t." I almost didn't graduate high school because I had skipped gym class so many times. Do you know my first impression with athletics and exercise? I used to go to my brother's Little League games, sit in the stands, and hear the parents, both mothers and fathers, screaming at the kids. Did you see the movie *Parenthood*, with Steve Martin? He was the coach of his son's Little League team. Do you recall the parents screaming from the stands at both the kids and the coach? That's what I am talking about. I remember parents screaming at their *own* kids when they made an error or struck out. So when my parents said, at the appropriate age, "Jim, would you like to play Little League?" my response was, "I don't think so." It wasn't until I was in London and began exercising on my own that I got over those early fears. Let's face it, there was no one to yell at me in Hyde Park or Kensington Gardens if I tripped or ran too slow; I chose not to play the tapes.

So think a moment. Once again explore your past and present relationship to food and exercise. There is a definite link between the two. I asked you to break that link, and you successfully did. Continuing this process will be necessary in order to continue to be a success in the weight-loss business. The old tapes will never be totally erased. You will simply respond to them differently and perhaps not play them so frequently.

Go back to your first thoughts regarding food. Did you think about food as a child? Were you considered athletic or nonathletic? This is especially appropriate for many women and overweight men who were immediately dismissed when it came to their athletic ability. I can't tell you the number of very fit, coordinated adults who are, to say the least, a little upset at their parents for never giving them a chance to explore their athletic ability. This is especially true for many women. I personally know one woman who had a contentious relationship with her mother surrounding the issue of athletic participation. She told me she wanted to run a marathon to prove to her mother, long deceased, and to herself, that she could do it. This was a triumph she needed to experience and a way for her to put some closure on the subject.

I recently went to my twentieth high school reunion. For those of you who've attended these functions, they really stir up past feelings regarding who you were at an earlier age. Once people heard what my profession was, I constantly heard the remark, "You're in *what* industry?" as people remembered how unathletic I had been in high school. My wife said, "Why do all these people keep saying this to you?" She met me when I was a fitness trainer. Even she does not realize this was a big change in my life—to consider myself an athletic, fit person. This was and still is an issue. And may I say, some of the formerly fit jocks and cheerleaders no longer appeared to be so fit.

YOU ARE NOW A DIFFERENT PERSON

This brings me to an observation. Over the years, I have had much better success professionally with people who have struggled with their weight all their lives than those individuals who never had to watch their weight and awake one day thirty pounds heavier. The early strugglers, myself included, always had to watch what they ate and are familiar with this often difficult, emotionally charged issue. But, hey, we're used to it. It is more a function of managing emotions, balancing diet and exercise, than anything else. The other group, those who made it through say thirty to forty years without ever having to think about what they ate, suddenly have a very difficult time when I ask them to explore their eating and exercise habits. I had a client for a very brief period of time who was very short, was forty-five years old, ate a croissant or Danish for breakfast, fries for lunch, and steak for dinner. No lie. Then, as you can well imagine, she started to gain weight. As I said, we only worked together for a brief period. Our relationship soured when I explained that she had been very lucky these past years to have been able to eat those types and quantities of food without gaining weight. But now her body had changed. She was older. She had lost lean muscle tissue and had never embraced a strength and resistance program. Frankly, she had never exercised, period. Her body could no longer handle these high-fat, high-calorie foods. She said if she exercised with me once a week, the weight would come off. I explained that was an unrealistic expectation. She chose to terminate my services.

This same phenomenon occurs in some businesses. For a period of time an industry may operate in one environment. Then, for whatever reason, government or increased competition may step in and suddenly the rules change. Either a company adapts to these new rules or, most likely, it faces huge penalties, loss of market share, decreased revenue, and possibly even be forced out of business. The same applies to your body. The rules change as you age. That I can guarantee. You can choose to adapt to the new set of rules, or you may find yourself "closed for business" sooner than you might have liked. Adaptation is necessary throughout one's life. And keep in mind, all adaptation need not be painful.

Okay, regardless of whether you have always had to be on plan or are a new participant, you are now an established success in your business venture: weight loss. How do others around you respond, and more important, how do you respond to yourself?

Let's start with you. If you've been on *The Business Plan for the Body,* you are now a different person. You have to accept that fact. You look better, feel better, and probably are more productive at your job or in your home. Every day it's a kick to get out of the shower, catch a glimpse of yourself, and think, "Not bad, not bad at all." I don't care what age you are. If you have succeeded at weight loss, done your strength and resistance training, improved your body composition and posture, you look better than ever. Period. Next, you bend down to get something out of a cabinet. Your back doesn't hurt, your knees don't ache. Everything you do in the morning seems easier. Why? Well, as I said before, your muscles are stronger, subsequently your joints don't ache. Your posture is better, so you don't overuse the lower back to perform simple tasks. Plus, you sleep better, and consequently are more rested when you get up in the morning. These are the great benefits derived from your hard work.

APPLY THE BPB PRINCIPLES TO OTHER ASPECTS OF YOUR LIFE

You most likely smile more, walk a little faster, carry yourself with more confidence. Whether you believe it or not, you're projecting a new energy, a very positive one at that. Remember what my friend Dick Walsh said: "The world gets out of the way for a man with a plan." You are that man, or woman, and you represent someone who clearly articulated a mission statement, did research, went public, assembled a management team, and followed through with your intent. You have a formula for success. Now you may decide to approach other areas of your life that you feel could profit from change. This could be your job, career satisfaction, your love life, or it could be as simple as deciding to take piano or skiing lessons, something you never thought you could successfully do. In other words, you took your mission statement—weight loss—and turned it into a reality. With that goal achieved, and the self-confidence that comes with achieving one's goal, why should you not fulfill all of your dreams and desires? You can do it. You've successfully done it with your weight and appearance, and the same principles apply to other aspects of your life that you would like to change. All you need is a plan.

For example, take an inventory of your physical appearance. Clearly you possess a new energy, and you definitely project a leaner, healthier visual. What about some of the other factors that relate to your appearance? Is it time to make a change? Do you need new clothes? Is it time for a new hairstyle? Could your teeth benefit from a long-delayed trip to the dentist? All these will complement your new, healthier visual. Start with your clothes. If your budget allows, buy some new clothes. Don't tailor the old ones to death. First of all, if you have lost a significant amount of weight, the old clothes will never look right if they have to be taken in so much. Second, those clothes represent the old you, not the new you. Now that you are thinner and in such better shape, you may notice the joy of throwing on jeans or khakis and a T-shirt, cotton shirt, or simple blouse.

THROW AWAY THE BODY CAMOUFLAGE

You don't need all that "camouflage" you used in the past to hide your weight, such as baggy skirts and dresses or pants and big tops. Enjoy tucking your shirt in. Adopting this style of dress is easy, low in cost, and really feels great. I do it all the time. Walk down the street. Look at the Banana Republic ads. Who looks good? Fit-looking individuals in simple, comfortable clothing. That's now you.

One of my long-term clients struggles with her weight but has really done a good job over the years. She is five-four, in her early fifties, and tries to keep her weight in the low 120s. She has tons of clothes. Her favorite outfit when she is down in weight—jeans, black cashmere sweater tucked in (that's the biggie, tucked in), belt, shoes, purse, done. And she looks great in it. She says when she can fit in the outfit, it makes her feel so good that it is all she wants to wear. You can do the same.

So buy some new clothing. Enjoy the experience. How about your hair? This is definitely the time to assess your hairstyle. Be open to suggestions from your stylist. Update. The same applies to men and facial hair. Many men grow beards to hide a double chin. You may decide the time has come to check out that chin. I bet you'll be shocked by what you see. You may decide to try a new hairstylist. Do a little research, just as we did in Chapter 2. Ask some friends. Stop people on the street who have great-looking hair. People love to be complimented and will often willingly give a referral. Make it fun. You deserve to treat yourself after all the hard work. All of these changes also continue to reinforce the fact that you are not going back to the old you. No way. You are not going to be one of those people who, briefly, looked great but then suffered a relapse. This is you, this is life, you did it.

What about your teeth? This is a personal favorite of mine. Take a look at people in the film and television industries. They have great teeth. Are they theirs? No, they clearly had work done, generally either having porcelain veneers or completely capping each tooth. Both of these options are very expensive, somewhere in the vicinity of five hundred to thousands of dollars a tooth. This might not be an option for you. What is an option is better dental care. Make sure to have your teeth cleaned twice a year. Don't be a baby about the dentist. When there, ask your dentist about a whitening option, which ranges in price, or some bonding of your teeth, which is less expensive than the other options I described. With bonding, which I have, slight imperfections are corrected with a bonding agent that hardens and becomes a part of the permanent tooth. It looks great. Or just whiten your teeth, which leads to a far more youthful appearance. Just like your health, weight, and appearance, correcting your teeth requires planning and some expense. Just approach it with intelligence. Make a plan. And just a side note on tooth care. Some studies show there is a correlation between decay in teeth and decline in physical health. Keep your mouth as healthy as your body. And remember the final word the old man gave to Meg Ryan and Alec Baldwin in the movie *Prelude to a Kiss:* floss!

There may be other factors about your appearance that have bothered you over the years. Just prioritize, look at the time, energy, and money involved, and decide what you want to do. My goal is not to make you feel there is anything wrong with your current appearance. Rather, my goal is to reinforce the fact that this is the *new* you.

Dealing with your emotions when it comes to your new energy and appearance is one issue. Preparing yourself to deal with how the rest of the world perceives the new you is yet another. Basically, you will encounter two distinct types of people once you succeed in the weight-loss business: the emotionally healthy and the emotionally unhealthy. Don't even for a moment think that I am talking about physical health; it's mental health all the way.

BE PREPARED FOR REACTIONS TO YOUR SUCCESS

Hopefully, you'll encounter far more of the emotionally healthy. These people are happy for you and your success. Some of these individuals may have been a part of your management team, or encouraged and praised you throughout the process. Others may just bump into you on the street after not seeing you for a few months and say, "You look great!" Be prepared, healthy people will make positive remarks to you like, "How did you do it?" Or, "You are giving me the courage to give weight loss a try." This praise is great for one's self-esteem.

Statements such as these reinforce your positive attitude and your proven ability to succeed. You must accept the fact that you become a role model for others when you achieve success in the weight-loss business. Go with that role. Share your experiences with others. By all means, recommend *The Business Plan for the Body*! I have met many people over the years who have been members of Weight Watchers. Many of the successful "losers" step into a leadership role with their Weight Watchers group. Some may check people in once a week at meetings, others may actually lecture on weight loss and weight-loss strategies. I really like this concept because, once again, taking a leadership role reinforces your ongoing success in the weight-loss business and your adherence to the plan. It additionally assists in keeping you focused on your weight-loss plan.

I know several people who have started their own weight-loss support group. These groups, similar to investment or book clubs, are for people who are in, or wish to be in, the weight-loss business. Whether an individual is in the embryonic stage of his or her plan or a proven success, all participants can benefit from fresh ideas, a new exercise, a great restaurant for "their" kind of food, or simply additional support to stay on plan. This group provides you with an environment you can revisit every week that sustains you in your plan. I have said all along, the plan grows and evolves with life. It is not a static plan. Use a group environment to explore how all participants can stay the course, and maintain the plan. Everyone benefits.

START YOUR OWN SUPPORT GROUP

Thus, mentally healthy people will make you feel great about yourself and your newfound success. But what about the emotionally unhealthy individuals you encounter? What should you expect from them?

Let me start with a story. I have changed the names to protect the guilty and the innocent. Years ago an overweight client, a "Mrs. Smith," referred another overweight woman, a "Mrs. Jones," to my firm. After about a year, Mrs. Smith had not lost weight, had not achieved her goal, and was struggling. Mrs. Jones, on the other hand, lost a great deal of weight, looked and felt terrific. I should mention that Mrs. Jones had been a chocoholic for many years and finally, through the assistance of my program, had overcome her obsession with chocolate. You will never guess what Mrs. Smith sent Mrs. Jones to congratulate her on her weight loss. You got it, a huge basket, probably well in excess of $100, of every conceivable type of chocolate. I remember sitting in Mrs. Jones's kitchen and looking at this "gift."

What I have just recounted is an example of a blatant hostile response. An additional personal favorite is the expression, "You're getting too thin." I have heard this comment hundreds of times over the years. I always say to clients, once you hear the "too thin" comment, know that you really are starting to look good. This remark is a clear passive-aggressive attempt to sabotage your weight loss. What your so-called friend is obviously saying is that they are threatened by your success in the weight-loss business. The person making the comment is insecure and unhappy with his or her own health, appearance, and body weight.

Please know this "too thin" comment applies to individuals who have lost weight in a healthy manner. This does not apply to anorexic or bulimic individuals who do become too thin as a result of the drastic measures they employ.

Next, you probably will hear the famous line, "You're obsessed with your eating and exercise." Yes, people will say to your face or mutter behind your back that you are obsessed. I get this comment all the time. My response to this comment is, "Where does an intelligent, well-devised, comprehensive health and weight-loss plan end and obsession begin?" I discussed this issue in Chapter 2, regarding being on plan part-time. You cannot be on plan part-time and realistically expect to achieve success. As I earlier said, you can't save then overspend, and expect to save money. Similarly, you can't show up for work part-time (unless, of course, it is a part-time job) and expect to be continually employed. You can't diet on the weekdays and relax on the weekends. This doesn't work! If at a birthday party someone is desperate for you to blow your diet and eat cake, tell a white lie and say you don't like chocolate or you have an upset stomach. Or just be honest and tell them you do not want the cake because you do not want to increase your daily caloric allocation. Explain how hard you have worked to achieve your present level of success. You don't want to backtrack. Usually that's enough to end the issue.

SUCCESSFUL PEOPLE ARE NOT OBSESSED, THEY ARE FOCUSED

Of course you can go ahead and eat the cake if you want it. Just know, for the rest of the day, you are going to have to be very careful if you want to stay on plan. Again, no food is a "no." Just make sure what you eat is accounted for and a part of your daily eating allocation.

You can tell, I get very irritated by certain situations and comments. My office is run by two other people: Bob, public relations and marketing, and Patti, who handles all our business affairs. Bob is fifty-eight, lifts weights four to five times a week, and is in great shape. Same for Patti, forty-nine, with a terrific figure; she actually was a fitness trainer before working with my firm. When the three of us are out at a party or some other social function, people actually make comments when junk food is around, such as, "I bet the three of you don't eat this," as if we've done something wrong by looking good and being in shape. Sure, we'll eat it if we want, but not because someone is challenging us to eat something we don't want or even like. We eat what makes us feel good and look good. That is our choice.

This is where the concept of corporate culture comes into play. My office culture is a healthy one, not because it is the nature of the business but because we want it that way. Keep in mind, there are a lot of overweight fitness trainers running around, but not at my firm. When the office has a monthly staff meeting, I order healthy food, such as turkey sandwiches, chicken skewers, or steamed chicken with vegetables and rice, and always include a big platter of fruit. I only got shot down once with my cheeseless pizza, which I was unanimously told was a bust (though grilled veggie pizza without cheese is one of my favorites). That is our culture. Our corporate culture also revolves around drinking water. We are all huge water drinkers and have to stop working every twenty to thirty minutes for a bathroom break.

CONTINUE TO CONTROL YOUR OFFICE AND HOME CULTURE

You may not realize it, but your home also has a corporate culture. How, what, and when you eat dictates that culture. To a certain extent your office is not in your control, but your home is definitely a place where you can call the shots regarding food. If friends are coming over for a Super Bowl party, serve some of their favorites, but include veggies, fruit, and other healthier choices so you don't go hungry or go off plan.

The Business Plan for the Body

If you are a guest at a similar party, volunteer to bring something you know you can eat and will keep you on plan. I do that all the time. Granted, you may get the "obsessive" or "food police" comment, but that is up to your friends. I can't change that. What I can help you change is your response to their comments. Don't be defensive. The nicer you are as a thin, healthy, attractive person—if you're nonjudgmental, nonconfrontational—the harder it will be for them to hate you because you are a success in the weight-loss business.

Be prepared for people to challenge your plan and beliefs on weight loss. I have had hundreds of people, quite overweight, look me in the eye and tell me I know nothing about diet, exercise, and weight loss. On one occasion I had to deal with an overweight (by at least fifty pounds) neurosurgeon at a pool party who challenged me for about an hour regarding my plan and weight-loss philosophy. About a dozen people listened with their mouths open. Finally, exasperated, I smiled politely and excused myself. Later, those who watched the exchange asked how I kept my cool. I explained, "It happens all the time. Overweight people constantly tell me their program is better than mine and challenge me on my beliefs." Would you go up to Ted Turner and tell him he knows nothing about cable news? Would you confront Bill Gates and tell him he knows nothing about the computer business? Would you tell Jerry Seinfeld he knows nothing about writing and starring in a television sitcom? Of course not. But when it comes to weight loss, everyone seems to be an expert. And since they are all experts, why are so many of them overweight? This is similar to attending a successful business seminar run by a bunch of CEOs whose companies are in bankruptcy.

REMEMBER, YOU RESEARCHED THE COMPETITION

Over 55 percent of all men and women in the United States, or 111 million, are overweight, so expect to provoke a strong response from people when the subject of weight or weight loss is discussed. Think about it. More than one out of every two people you come in contact with shares your *need* to lose weight, but only a few actually attempt to act on that need. The question remains: How many people will be happy for you and how many will be jealous, either consciously or subconsciously? I don't mean to belabor this issue, but I don't want you to be caught off guard, unprepared, and hurt by the responses you receive. This is not easy. Actually, this may be harder than the plan itself. Just be happy, be clear, stay focused. You have succeeded where others have failed. It's your life, not theirs.

Your friends and colleagues knew you before *The Business Plan for the Body*. We have explored many of their likely responses to your weight-loss success. But you should also be prepared for the new people whom you meet and make comments such as, "I bet you were always thin," or, "You look like the type who can just eat anything." Be very direct and say, "I wish that were the case but it isn't. I am on plan. I used to be heavier and out of shape. I struggle with it all the time." Say it, because you and I know it's the truth. I keep using myself as an example, but people constantly think that I have always been in this shape. As I told you, that could not be further from the truth. I am on plan, and I'm going to be on plan, for the rest of my life. I don't intend on ever retiring from my business venture, at least not until I am ultimately "retired." Nor should you.

ALWAYS BE HONEST ABOUT YOUR ONGOING STRUGGLE

There are many things in life we can imagine and accomplish, others we can't. One goal definitely within your power is improving your body, health, and appearance. No one can make you eat something. Nothing should keep you from exercising, unless you allow it. I just don't buy the excuse "I don't have time." Yes you do. You find time for those things in life that you really desire to do. You just have to do some restructuring of your day, or ask your spouse, friend, or family member, or hire someone, to help make it happen. Close your eyes and imagine what you could look and feel like. Then make it happen.

The title to this chapter—"I Did It, I Did It"—is a direct quote from my daughter, Olivia. When she was two, she used to want help getting up onto our bed. We have a high sleigh bed that rests on a platform. Olivia would raise her hands up and say, "Daddy help, Daddy help." I would show her how she could get up on the bed herself by putting one foot on the platform and pulling on the sheets with her hands. She would struggle, sometimes cry, but then one day she got up on her own. Of course, you know what she said when she ultimately achieved her goal. That's right, she threw up her hands, jumped up and down, and cried, "I did it, I did it!" All she needed was a little help, some instruction, encouragement, and the determination to achieve her goal. My goal as a parent is for her to feel that regardless of the challenges she faces throughout her life, she will seek instruction, try as best as she can, persevere, and ultimately be able to say, "I did it, I did it."

I believe in her ability to accomplish anything to which she sets her mind. Of course, as her parent I'm biased. But stop for one moment and think about yourself. How many times in your life have you thrown up your hands and cried, "I did it, I did it"? Remember how **YOU DID IT,** great that sense of accomplishment felt? I hope **YOU DID IT.** this journey we have taken produced one of those times. I hope that I have given you the road map and the tools to become a smashing success in the weight-loss business. I hope almost every day you think about your plan, your continued success, and even if only to yourself, take a brief moment and say, "I did it, I did it."

RESOURCE NOTES

INTRODUCTION
The New England Journal of Medicine, 1998

CHAPTER 1
Consumer Reports on Health, January 2000
FDA Consumer, Health Responsibility Systems, Inc.

CHAPTER 2
Calorie Control Council, from the Internet @
Caloriecontrol.org./index.html
Chicago Tribune, October 27, 1999; Bob Condor, February 13, 2000;
April 5, 2000, Section 5
Consumer Reports on Health, June 1992
Environmental Nutrition, February, March, April 2000
Fumento, Michael, *The Fat of the Land Obesity Epidemic* (Viking Penguin Press), excerpted from The American Enterprise Institute for Public Policy Research, September 1997
Health (magazine), April 1999
Johns Hopkins Medical Letter, May 2000, Vol. 12, Issue 3
Journal of the American Medical Association, October 27, 1999
Newsweek (magazine), Special Issue, Spring/Summer 1999
New York Times News Service, May 9, 2000
Shape (magazine), April 2000
Tufts University Health & Nutrition Letter, March 1997, Vol. 15, No. 1, and August 1998, Vol. 16, No. 6
University of California at Berkeley Wellness Newsletter, June 1996
W (magazine), April 4, 2000

CHAPTER 3
Health magazine

CHAPTER 4
The Wall Street Journal, December 28, 1999

CHAPTER 5

Colorado State University Cooperative Extension, February 28, 1998
Consumer Reports on Health, January 1992
Environmental Nutrition, February 2000
Health, April & October 1999, March & April 2000
IDEA Personal Trainer, April 2000
Journal of the American Medical Association, 1998
Nutritional Basics Home Page, from the Internet, excerpted from the
    AMA Complete Guide to Women's Health, December 2, 1998
Windy City Sports, March 1999

CHAPTER 6

Consumer Reports on Health, November 1999, January 2000
Environmental Nutrition, December 1996, October 1999
Fumento, Michael, *The Fat of the Land*
Health, April 1999, March 1999, March 2000
Nutrition Action Newsletter, July/August 1999
Parade (magazine), October 22, 1989
Shape, February 2000
Tufts University Health & Nutrition Letter, June 1997, October 1998,
    September 1999
U.S. News & World Report, January 8, 1996

CHAPTER 7

American Health, April 13, 1994
AOL News Profiles @ AOL.net.
Colorado State Cooperative Extension, "Lifting Weights Reduces
    Weight," Barbara Martin, February 26, 1998
Consumer Reports on Health, December 1995, June 1999, January
    2000
Environmental Nutrition, September 1993
Health, January/February 2000
Nelson, Miriam E., *Strong Women Stay Thin* (Bantam Books), 1997
Newsweek, August 2, 1999 & July 19, 2000
Nutrition Action Newsletter, September 1996
Resource Manual for Guidelines for Exercise Testing and Prescription,
    2nd edition
Shape, February 2000
Time, February 28, 2000
Tufts University Health & Nutrition Letter, May 1999 & October 1995
University of Texas Lifetime Health Letter, Vol. 4, No. 2
U.S. News & World Report, January 8, 1996
Virtual Resources (from the Internet)

CHAPTER 8

Chicago Tribune Magazine, March 26, 2000
Consumer Reports on Health, January 2000
Mayo Clinic Health Letter, July 2000
More (magazine), January/February 1999
Nutrition Action Newsletter, July/August 1999

CHAPTER 9

Shape, July 2000

INDEX

A

abdominals (exercises), 152
abdominals (muscles), 186
abductor muscles, 149
activity multipliers, 62–63, 91
    and staying on weight-loss
        program, 178, 180
    weight-loss goal setting
        and, 161
adolescents, 68
    see also children
adrenaline, 78
aerobics instructors, 2–3
age, aging, 5, 13–14, 89
    exercise and, 111, 113–14,
        118–19, 129
    and fallacies about weight-
        loss dieting, 35–36, 41
    and fruits and vegetables,
        20
    slowing process of, 14, 20
    and staying on weight-loss
        program, 176–77, 180
    weight-loss success and,
        204
    see also elderly
Agriculture Department, U.S.
    (USDA), 93–94
    Agricultural Research
        Service of, 93

food pyramid of, 99
Human Nutrition Research
    Center on Aging of, 89
on labeling, 30
airline food, 197
alcohol, 85
    eating allocation and,
        104–5
    and staying on weight-loss
        program, 199–200
allocation:
    definition of, 82–83
    see also eating allocation
American College of Sports
    Medicine, 21, 122
American Dietetic
    Association (ADA), 21,
        101–2
American Heart Association,
    120
American Medical
    Association, 65–66
    on exercise, 112–13
amino acids, 66
amphetamines, 74
anterior deltoids, 153
antibodies, 66
antidepressant drugs, 92, 165
antioxidants, 77
anti-sugar diets, 22–23

apples, apple pie, 94
Archway Fat-Free Devil's
    Food Cookies, 29
arthritis, 14, 118-19
asparagus, 93
asthma, 103
Atkins diet, 19

B
back, 153
    lower, *see* lower back
    strength and resistance
        training for, 138-39
back extensions, 150
back rows, 139
bad breath, 20, 103
bad days, 40-41
bad lunches, 90
bagels, 99, 194
baked potatoes, 99, 195
balsamic vinegar, 30
basal metabolic rates (BMRs),
    61-64, 73-74, 76-78
    eating allocation and, 91
    exercise and, 109, 122, 127
    progression and, 189
    and staying on weight-loss
        program, 174, 177-79
    weight-loss goal setting
        and, 159, 161
beans, 66, 94
beer, light, 199
behavior:
    and fallacies about weight-
        loss dieting, 27-28
    metabolism and, 65, 68-70,
        75, 78
    and staying on weight-loss
        program, 199

weight-loss intentions and,
    49
Benedict, Francis G., 61
bicep curls, 183, 185
    sitting on the ball, 144
biceps, 144, 182-83, 185
bicycling, 111, 113, 127-28,
    131
    progression and, 190-92
big-boned, 36-37
big events, 196-97
binging, 40-41, 166
    eating allocation and,
        91-92, 96
bio impedance, 169
blood sugar, 119-20
blood type programs, 23
body:
    challenging it to change,
        34
    plateauing of, 33-34
    structural integrity of, 121,
        153-55
body fat, 37, 181
    definition of, 60
    eating allocation and, 83
    exercise and, 122-23
    and fallacies about weight-
        loss dieting, 33
    measurement of, 168-70
    metabolism and, 60, 64,
        66-68, 73
    and staying on weight-loss
        program, 174, 180
    weight-loss goal setting
        and, 160, 168-70
    weight-loss intentions and,
        47
    see also fat, fats
body language, 9, 14-15

body pump classes, 184
body type programs, 23
bones, bone mineral density, 66
  exercise and, 119–21, 127
brain:
  current weight-loss diets and, 20
  increasing blood flow to, 14
bread, breads, 66–67, 94–96, 194, 196
  eating allocation and, 95–96, 98–99
breakfasts:
  eating allocation and, 95–96
  and staying on weight-loss program, 194, 196
  weight-loss success and, 204
  weight-loss support and, 56–57
breathing, 137
bridging on the ball, 151
broccoli, 18, 42, 93
brownies, 198
Brown University, Weight Control and Diabetes Research Center at, 195
buffets, 173
  eating allocation and, 101–2, 106
  and staying on weight-loss program, 196
bulking up, 122
Burger King, 97
business dinners, 195
business plans, 1, 4–5, 11
butter, 99

C
Caesar salads, 85–86, 197
caffeine:
  eating allocation and, 104
  metabolism and, 74, 77–78
cake, cakes, 40, 89, 100, 165, 209–10
calcium, 19
calipers, 169–70
caloric awareness, 87–88, 92, 106
caloric deficit, 30, 39–41, 117
  and staying on weight-loss program, 174, 180–81
  weight-loss goal setting and, 162
caloric density, 89–90
calories, 1, 3–4, 18, 59–68, 81–107, 156, 161–66
  current weight-loss diets and, 20, 22–25
  definition of, 60
  eating allocation and, 83–107
  exercise and, 108–9, 111, 113–18, 122
  and fallacies about weight-loss dieting, 26, 28–32, 34–35, 38–41
  liquid, see liquid calories
  metabolism and, 60–68, 70–77, 91
  progression and, 177, 181–82, 185, 189–90, 192, 200
  and staying on weight-loss program, 173–74, 177–81, 194–99
  weight-loss goal setting and, 158–59, 161–64, 166

heart, heart disease, *see* cardiovascular system, cardiovascular disease
heart rate monitors, 115, 135, 155, 190
heart rates:
exercise and, 112, 114–16, 131, 133
progression and, 184–85, 190–91
high blood pressure, 14
exercise and, 120
and fallacies about weight-loss dieting, 31, 38
stimulants and, 74
high-fat, high-calorie treats, 95–98
highly restrictive low-calorie diets, 67
high-protein, low-carbohydrate diets, 25, 98, 160
high-protein diets, 19–21, 49, 66, 94, 159
hip abduction, 149
hip extensions, 134, 148
hips, 41–42
hormones, 28, 66, 70–71, 78, 122
hors d'oeuvres, 173
eating allocation and, 101–2, 106
and staying on weight-loss program, 195–96
hydrostatic weighing, 168–70
hypothyroidism, 70

I
ice cream, 29–30, 101
ice skating, 111

immune system, 20, 25
injuries:
exercise and, 32–33, 118, 121–22, 132, 153–55, 166, 183–84
progression and, 183–84, 191
insulin, 22, 33, 66, 120
intestines, 25
Italian food, 85, 98

J
jalapeño peppers, 78
joints:
exercise and, 118–19, 183–84
and fallacies about weight-loss dieting, 33, 35
progression and, 183–84, 190–93
weight-loss success and, 205
juice, 105–6
junk food, 198, 210

K
Karas, Jim:
education of, 1, 13, 62
typical food diary entry of, 96
ketosis, 20, 49, 159
kidneys, kidney stones, 19, 25, 103
Kraft Fat-Free Ranch Dressing, 29

physical appearance, 9–10
    of author, 13
    exercise and, 120
    weight-loss success and,
        201–2, 205–7, 209–12
    weight-loss support and,
        56
physical fitness:
    current weight-loss diets
        and, 26
    exercise and, 110, 112–14
    and fallacies about weight-
        loss dieting, 33, 35
    mission statements and,
        11–12
    overweight and, 33
    weight-loss success and,
        206, 210
    weight-loss support and, 56
pizza, 198
    cheeseless, 210
    weight-loss support and,
        55
polyunsaturated fat, 23, 30,
    66
Pondimin, 74
popcorn, 94
posture:
    exercise and, 120, 127,
        136–37, 154–55
    weight-loss success and,
        205
potato chips, 89, 95, 165, 198
potatoes, 66, 97–99, 195–96
    French fries and, 93,
        97–98, 198
    mashed, 93, 165, 196
poultry, 54, 66, 210
    eating allocation and,
        94–95, 99

and staying on weight-loss
    program, 196–97
pressure, 46, 49
prioritizing, 164
Pritikin, Nathan, 23–24
*Pritikin Program for Diet &
    Exercise, The* (Pritikin),
    23–24
productivity, 14
progression:
    cardiovascular exercise
        and, 182, 184–85,
        189–92
    exercise and, 115, 123,
        125, 128–29, 133, 135,
        153, 177, 182–93
    methods of, 182–89
    misconceptions regarding,
        192–93
    and staying on weight-loss
        program, 177, 181–82,
        193–200
    and strength and resistance
        training, 71–72, 182–93
protein, proteins:
    current weight-loss diets
        and, 19–22, 25
    eating allocation and, 94,
        98, 101, 106
    metabolism and, 65–68
    weight-loss goal setting
        and, 159–60
    weight-loss intentions and,
        49
Prozac, 92
push-ups, 142

Q
quadriceps, 153, 186

sodium (*cont.*):
    and staying on weight-loss
        program, 197
    weight-loss goal setting
        and, 159–60
soreness, pain vs., 192–93
soup, 104
specificity, 128
spicy food, 78
spinach, 93
spin classes, 184
spouses, 49–53
    exercise and, 130
    and staying on weight-loss
        program, 198
    weight-loss intentions and,
        49
    weight-loss support and,
        50–53, 55–56, 58
Spri, *see* exercise tubing
spritzers, 199
squats, 145, 185
stairclimbing, StairMasters,
    108, 111–12, 115, 117,
    131, 133
    progression and, 190–92
standing exercise, posture for,
    136
standing lateral raises, 141
starches, 66
starvation:
    metabolism and, 67–68
    weight-loss goal setting
        and, 165
stationary bikes, 108, 111–12,
    117–18, 133
stationary lunges, 146
step classes, 184
Stillman diet, 19
stimulants, 74–76, 78

strength and resistance train-
    ing, 13, 24, 108–14,
    117–29
adding instability to,
    186–88, 191
allocating time for,
    130–33, 155, 182, 189
benefits of, 111, 118–21
building and executing
    periodization program
    for, 187–89
changing angle in, 185–87
changing equipment in, 187
comparisons between car-
    diovascular exercise and,
    111–12, 118, 127
essential components of,
    128–29
exercise equipment for,
    125, 138–41, 143–44,
    151–53
and fallacies about weight-
    loss dieting, 35–38
imbalances corrected by,
    154
increasing number of sets
    in, 184–88
and metabolism, 71–73,
    75–76
and muscle, 37, 71–72
program for, 138–54
and progression, 71–72,
    182–93
proper breathing for, 137
questions and common
    misconceptions regard-
    ing, 121–29
reducing speed in, 185–87
repetitions in, 123–25, 128,
    133–34, 153

ABOUT THE AUTHOR

JIM KARAS is a graduate of the Wharton School of Business, attended the London School of Economics, worked as a highly successful private portfolio manager, and created Solo Sessions, the most successful weight-loss management firm in Chicago. In addition to lecturing and presenting workshops, he has been featured on ABC's *Good Morning America*. Jim resides in Chicago with his wife, Ellen, and their two children, Olivia and Evan.